I Will

LOSE WEIGHT

THIS TIME!

DIET JOURNAL

Includes

100 HELPFUL TIPS

for **WEIGHT-LOSS**

Alex Lluch

I WILL LOSE WEIGHT THIS TIME! DIET JOURNAL

BY ALEX LLUCH

Nutritional and fitness guidelines based on information provided by the Uni
States Food and Drug Administration, Food and Nutrition Information Cen
National Agricultural Library, Agricultural Research Service, and the U
Department of Agriculture.

Cover Image: Sandals, the Caribbean's #1 Ultra All-inclusive Resorts
Photo courtesy of Sandals Resorts

ISBN-13: 978-1-887169-55-4
ISBN-10: 1-887169-55-5

Printed in China

TABLE OF CONTENTS

INTRODUCTION 5

HOW TO USE THIS DIET JOURNAL 7

OTHER GREAT FEATURES OF THIS DIET JOURNAL 11
- "Away-From-Home" Mini Diet Journal 11
- Your Weight-Loss Progress Chart 11
- Nutrition Facts on Popular Food Items 12

ASSESSING YOUR WEIGHT & HEALTH STATUS 13
- Body Mass Index - BMI 14
- Is Your Weight a Health Risk? 15
- Identify Your Eating Patterns 16

DEVELOPING A SUCCESSFUL WEIGHT-LOSS PROGRAM 17

THINGS YOU SHOULD KNOW TO LOSE WEIGHT 21
- Suggested Daily Calories for Weight Maintenance 21
- Suggested Daily Calories for Weight-Loss 21
- Recommended Daily Amount From Each Food Group 22
- How Many Servings Should I Eat? 22
- A Handy Measuring System 23
- Water Works Wonders 23
- The Nutrition Facts Label 24
- Label At-A-Glance 24
- A Breakdown of the Nutrition Facts Label 25
- What Are the Different Types of Fats? 28
- Best Sources for Essential Nutrients 29
- Dietary Guidelines for Americans 30
- Exercise for Fitness and Fun 31
- A Complete Physical Fitness Program 32

TABLE OF CONTENTS

- Incorporate Activities Into Your Daily Routine 33
- Walking 34
- Health Benefits of Physical Activity 34
- Exercise and Weight Control 35
- Calories Burned for Typical Physical Activities 36

YOUR PERSONAL PROFILE... 39

**YOUR PERSONAL WEIGHT-LOSS GOALS,
PLANS, & ACHIEVEMENTS**... 43

THE SECRET TO WEIGHT-LOSS:
Keeping Track of What You Eat 51

DAILY NUTRITIONAL INTAKE & GOALS ACHEIVED 56

NUTRITIONAL FACTS ON POPULAR FOOD ITEMS 259

INTRODUCTION

BY PURCHASING THIS BOOK, YOU HAVE TAKEN THE FIRST STEP in your weight-loss journey to looking and feeling great. Whether you are a veteran of the diet game, or in search of a comprehensive weight-loss program, this is the right book for you!

More than half of American adults today are overweight, with one-third considered obese. America's weight problem has become a serious issue because of the increasing number of diseases linked to being overweight, such as high cholesterol, high blood pressure, diabetes, stroke, and heart disease. Such diseases can reduce the quality of life and, in some cases, lead to death. In America, obesity causes roughly 300,000 deaths each year, while healthcare costs of adults who are obese continue to rise. Several factors can contribute to being overweight, including family genetics, the growing portion sizes of food, and the tendency to overeat. The most common way to determine whether or not a person is obese is through Body Mass Index, or BMI. This is a ratio of a person's height and weight, and when a person's BMI is over 25, he or she can be considered overweight. Unfortunately, BMIs over 25 are an increasing trend in America's health statistics. We are a nation whose waistline is expanding, and will continue to grow unless we take control of our eating and exercise habits.

Losing weight has major benefits that can improve your way of life. Weight -loss can lower the risk of the diseases mentioned above, help you become healthy and more active, and also make you look and feel better about yourself. It is difficult in today's society to make the right choices regarding your health and diet. Food portions in restaurants are larger, which encourage us to eat more; our jobs promote sedentary lifestyles; and fast food, while often unhealthy, is convenient and inexpensive. Many food companies use larger sized portions as selling points, making the claim that bigger is better. It then becomes the consumer's responsibility to monitor how much he or she eats and to know how much is personally enough. That is where this journal comes in: it educates you on proper weight management and weight-loss methods. It provides important dietary and health information, and it helps you make the right decisions to begin your weight-loss plan so you can uncover a healthier, better-looking you!

By using this diet journal, you are taking charge of your weight-loss program. It is a useful resource of nutritional information and fitness guidelines and will help you assess your current weight and health status. Another advantage of this book is that it will guide you in setting down an appropriate plan for yourself. It also makes counting calories and keeping track of nutritional values simple.

Being aware of what you eat is an important step in the direction of weight-loss: it keeps you responsible for everything you consume, creating an on-going awareness of your diet program. When you write down everything you eat, you hold yourself accountable for your food consumption, so not even the tiniest bite of a cookie should slip by!

In addition, this journal will help you keep track of your daily progress as you move closer towards your weight-loss goal. This on-going routine will make your program more effective. With this journal as your companion, you can make better, more informed choices that will help you lose weight, look better, and improve your health! Congratulations!

HOW TO USE THIS DIET JOURNAL

Each section of this diet journal is specifically designed to help guide you through the various stages of your weight-loss program. It will allow you to assess your current health, identify eating behaviors and patterns that may prevent you from losing weight, provide proper nutrition and fitness guidelines, and help you create realistic goals and expectations as you go through your journey to look better and improve your health.

ASSESSING YOUR WEIGHT & HEALTH STATUS

Before you begin your quest, it is imperative to define your starting point, as well as your final goal. You can calculate your current status in height, weight, and Body Mass Index (BMI), and assess your health risks based on your genetic predisposition and family history. You should also investigate behaviors that may have led to your current weight situation, such as emotional triggers, guilt-based eating, and stress snacking.

DEVELOPING A SUCCESSFUL WEIGHT-LOSS PROGRAM

When developing your personal weight-loss program, you should keep in mind five main concepts: Motivation, Realistic Timelines, Personal Success, Visualization, and Maintenance. Reflecting on these essential points will help you determine the program that is individualized for your needs. Once you have defined these terms in relation to your own goals, you can establish additional habits that will assist you on your weight-loss journey.

Writing in your diet journal should become part of your daily routine. Be sure to take full advantage of your program by documenting the foods and beverages you consume in your journal. This way you will be able to stay motivated and keep track of your daily calorie allowance, nutritional value intake, and weight-loss progress.

THINGS YOU SHOULD KNOW TO LOSE WEIGHT

Nutritional Guidelines: Any successful weight-loss program should start with a full understanding of nutritional guidelines. Nutrition is a multi-faceted concept that includes a wide range of elements. Start your program armed with information on the USDA Food Guide, the Nutrition Facts label, average serving sizes, portion sizes, and the importance of drinking water.

This book will help you become an expert on food facts. Included in this journal are nutritional values for over 1,000 popular food items. This information will help you break down the nutritional content of the foods you eat during your diet. You will learn how to count calories and determine how sugar, sodium, cholesterol, carbohydrates, fats, and protein affect your body. By using this book, you will shed those unwanted pounds and be on your way to improved health.

Physical Activity: Burning calories through physical activity is a great way to expedite a successful weight-loss program. There are three points to consider in your overall weight-loss plan. The first is to select aerobic activities that will improve your body's metabolism and burn unwanted fat. You will learn how to analyze your lifestyle activities that burn calories, such as gardening or home maintenance. The second point is to start a strength-training program at the gym, or create your own home gym with a few affordable types of equipment like hand weights and exercise videos. The third point is to gently guide your body through a daily stretching routine and watch your flexibility improve. Physical activities can transform your body to a higher level of fitness and help you feel great.

YOUR PERSONAL PROFILE

Fill out your personal health profile at the start of your diet so you can accurately assess your current physical state, habits, and eating patterns. Documenting this information will assist you in identifying the areas of your diet and health that need improvement. If in doubt, consult with a professional so you can receive medical clearance to begin a safe diet and fitness program.

YOUR PERSONAL WEIGHT-LOSS GOALS, PLANS, & ACHIEVEMENTS

In this section, you will solidify your weight-loss goals and plans. You will be able to write down the specific targets you want to reach and the means you will take to achieve them. Be sure to establish realistic weight-loss goals that are broken down into daily, weekly, and monthly objectives.

You will also be able to document your results at the end of your program. Keep in mind that consistent effort and steady progress will help you achieve your target weight. You will be amazed at your weight-loss progress, reduced body-fat percentage, and new measurements. Take "before" and "after" photos to visually document your successful efforts.

THE SECRET TO WEIGHT-LOSS: Keeping Track of What You Eat

This section is the heart of your program because it is crucial to your weight-loss success. It is a source of personal feedback and a comprehensive daily reminder of all of the elements of your weight-loss plan. Your daily journal can help you stay focused on your personal goals and keep you motivated towards your weight-loss target. These pages will help you keep track of your food and beverage intake, make sure you are within your daily calorie allotment, and ensure that you are getting enough fluids. You will also be able to log your physical fitness activities, supplements, energy levels, and daily weight.

OTHER GREAT FEATURES OF THIS DIET JOURNAL

"AWAY FROM HOME" MINI DIET JOURNAL

Any time you are away from your home environment, simply slip your mini diet journal into your purse, jacket, or pocket and take it with you wherever you go. This is a convenient way to remain committed to your weight-loss program. You will stay on course by effectively recording the food and beverages you consume during your daily routine, whether at work, school, or while performing any other activities. When you return home, you can transfer the information to your diet journal and calculate the amount of calories, fat, carbs, etc., you have consumed. You should feel proud that you are using both your at-home and on-the-go diet journals, which will help you to achieve your weight-loss goals.

YOUR WEIGHT-LOSS PROGRESS CHART

Chart your daily, weekly, and/or monthly progress as you gradually achieve your weight-loss goals. This is an exciting way to map your progress towards a new and healthier you. It's also a way to build momentum and celebrate your success.

Customize the chart according to your personal weight-loss goals. Begin by recording your current weight in the far left column where it states "Start Here/Enter Weight." This marker provides enough space above and below your current weight to allow for fluctuation.

The horizontal lines of the graph signify pounds of weight. Decide how many pounds each horizontal line should indicate. For example, if you have a lot of weight to lose, you will probably want each horizontal line to indicate one pound. So if your starting weight is 170, you would write this down next to "Start Here/Enter Weight." If you want to lose 20 pounds, you would use each line to mark one pound of weight. Proceed to fill in the rest of the numbers on the left column. The line directly under your current weight would be 169 and would decrease until you reach your goal weight of 150. The lines above your current weight would start with 171 and up, to allow for fluctuation.

For moderate weight-loss, use every other line to record each pound. If you only have a minimal amount of weight to lose, you can use the dark-blue horizontal lines to indicate one pound.

The vertical lines indicate days of the week. You have the option of plotting your progress on a daily, weekly, or monthly basis. Each dark blue vertical line indicates the first day of each week. To chart your progress, simply locate the vertical line at the bottom of the page that corresponds to the day of your program. Follow the line until you reach your weight for the day on the left column. Mark that point. Repeat for each day or week of your program. As you progress through your program, connect the points to create a visual graph of your weight-loss.

NUTRITIONAL FACTS ON POPULAR FOOD ITEMS

This section is a great resource of nutritional information on foods you may want to select for your weight-loss program. It provides calories per serving as well as nutritional content for fat, protein, carbohydrates, and fiber. To use this section, look up food items listed in alphabetical order. Locate the corresponding information, and log the data into your journal so you can keep track of your daily totals.

ASSESSING YOUR WEIGHT
& HEALTH STATUS

The most important reasons to start a weight-loss program are to look and feel great, as well as reduce the risk of health complications, such as heart disease and diabetes. Before you start, however, it is important to assess your health status. There are three methods to determine your overall physical condition: your height and weight measurements, waist size, and Body Mass Index (BMI). Another consideration is your family history.

For adults 18 years and older, the first step is to measure your height and weight. Use those two numbers to find your BMI on the following page. If your BMI falls within the range of 19 to 24, you are considered healthy. If your BMI lands from 24 to 29, then you are at increased risk of developing health problems. If your BMI is 30 or above, you could be considered obese. If you fall into the last two categories, it is essential to plan and manage your weight-loss program.

The second factor in evaluating your weight is your waist size. Use a tape measure to calculate your waist circumference below your rib cage and above your belly button. You have an increased health risk for developing serious chronic illness if your waist size is more than 35 inches for women and 40 inches for men. For more information, see the chart on page 15.

Your personal history and family background can shed additional light on possible health risks. Be aware of increased potential problems if your family history includes arthritis, high blood pressure, high cholesterol, high blood sugar, death at a young age, heart problems, cancer, or respiratory illness. A history of family illness doesn't mean these conditions are destined to be a part of your future, but is yet another reason to get started on the road to good health and physical fitness.

BODY MASS INDEX - BMI

Body composition can vary greatly from individual to individual. Two people who possess the same height and weight can have different bone structure and varying percentages of muscle and fat. Therefore, your weight alone is not the only factor in assessing your risk for weight related health issues. Your BMI can help indicate whether or not your health is at risk.

Calculating your BMI: Locate your height in the left hand column below. Then move across the row to your weight. The number at the very top of the column is your BMI.

BMI	19	20	21	22	23	24	25	26	27	28	29	30	31	32	33	34	35
Height							**weight in pounds**										
4'10"	91	96	100	105	110	115	119	124	129	134	138	143	148	153	158	162	167
4'11"	94	99	104	109	114	119	124	128	133	138	143	148	153	158	163	168	173
5'	97	102	107	112	118	123	128	133	138	143	148	153	158	163	158	174	179
5'1"	100	106	111	116	122	127	132	137	143	148	153	158	164	169	174	180	185
5'2"	104	109	115	120	126	131	136	142	147	153	158	164	169	175	180	186	191
5'3"	107	113	118	124	130	135	141	146	152	158	163	169	175	180	186	191	197
5'4"	110	116	122	128	134	140	145	151	157	163	169	174	180	186	192	197	204
5'5"	114	120	126	132	138	144	150	156	162	168	174	180	186	192	198	204	210
5'6"	118	124	130	136	142	148	155	161	167	173	179	186	192	198	204	210	216
5'7"	121	127	134	140	146	153	159	166	172	178	185	191	198	204	211	217	223
5'8"	125	131	138	144	151	158	164	171	177	184	190	197	203	210	216	223	230
5'9"	128	135	142	149	155	162	169	176	182	189	196	203	209	216	223	230	236
5'10"	132	139	146	153	160	167	174	181	188	195	202	209	216	222	229	236	243
5'11"	136	143	150	157	165	172	179	186	193	200	208	215	222	229	236	243	250
6'	140	147	154	162	169	177	184	191	199	206	213	221	228	235	242	250	258
6'1"	144	151	159	166	174	182	189	197	204	212	219	227	235	242	250	257	265
6'2"	148	155	163	171	179	186	194	202	210	218	225	233	241	249	256	264	272
6'3"	152	160	168	176	184	192	200	208	216	224	232	240	248	256	264	272	279
		Healthy					**Overweight**						**Obese**				

IS YOUR WEIGHT A HEALTH RISK?

For most adults, BMI and waist size are relatively reliable ways to indicate whether or not you are overweight. These two indicators are also effective in assessing your risk of weight related health issues.

Your waist measurement determines whether or not you have the tendency to carry fat around your midsection. A higher waist size may indicate a greater risk for weight related health issues such as high blood pressure, Type 2 diabetes and coronary artery disease. Typically, the higher your Body Mass Index, the greater risk to your health. This risk also increases if your waist is greater than 35 inches for women or 40 inches for men.

If your weight indicates that you are at a higher risk for health problems, consult your primary care physician to determine safe and effective ways to improve your health. Even moderate amounts of weight-loss, around 5-10 percent of your weight, can have long lasting health benefits as long as you keep off the pounds.

Risk of Associated Disease According to BMI and Waist Size

Body Mass Index		Waist less than or equal to 40" Men 35" Women	Waist greater than 40" Men 35" Women
18 or less	Underweight	N/A	N/A
19-24	Normal	N/A	N/A
25-29	Overweight	Increased	High
30-35	Obese	High	Very High
over 35	Obese	Very High	Very High

IDENTIFY YOUR EATING PATTERNS

Changing your eating habits requires adjusting your attitude toward food. Begin by understanding the situations and emotional triggers that lead to overeating. Let's take a look at some common behaviors:

Are you compelled to eat as an emotional response to your thoughts and feelings? If you eat when you're upset, frustrated, angry, lonely, or tired, the answer most likely is yes. Food feels like the perfect temporary solution – that is, until it is finished, and then guilt sets in because the food choice may not have been healthy. Try to choose other behaviors as an emotional response, such as taking a walk or calling a friend.

Do you eat when you are not hungry because you think you should? Sometimes the time of day is enough encouragement to eat a meal or a quick snack, despite a lack of actual physical hunger. Instead, learn to listen to your body. If you are not hungry, you shouldn't eat.

Do you feel guilty leaving food on your plate? Perhaps when you were a child, you were told to finish all of the food on your plate. This sense of guilt should no longer gauge how much food you should eat. It is acceptable to stop eating when you feel full.

Do you make poor food choices because of peer pressure? It is far easier to go with the flow when those around you are eating unhealthy foods. It takes self-control and determination to follow your weight-loss plan at social gatherings or all-you-can-eat buffets. Congratulate yourself when you stick to your plan and successfully fend off unhealthy snacking urges.

Do you eat out of boredom? Food can become a time-filler when you are bored. Don't fall into this trap! Try to motivate yourself and choose a fun and interesting activity as an alternative to snacking. If you are otherwise occupied with an activity where food is not involved, it will be easier to wait for your regularly scheduled meal.

DEVELOPING A SUCCESSFUL
WEIGHT-LOSS PROGRAM

PERSONAL SUCCESS

Reaching your personal goals for your weight-loss program starts with the desire for success. As you move through each phase of your plan, the definition of success can take on many different meanings. In the previous chapter, success could be found in honestly assessing your weight and health status. Now is the time to fine-tune your personal interpretation of success by defining how the following key points can help you achieve your weight-loss goal.

Motivation: Your journey takes on a new challenge as you look at the reasons behind your desire for personal success. The first component is to discover your source of motivation. What are your top three reasons for pursuing your weight-loss goal? Write them down in this journal and read them often as a reminder and a source of inspiration. They will help you stay focused on your future weight-loss goals.

Realistic Timelines: The second component is to set realistic goals for yourself. Select a healthy plan and allow an appropriate length of time for your program to succeed. Promises of quick weight-loss may sound too good to be true and most likely are unhealthy and possibly dangerous. General guidelines for healthy weight-loss suggest losing 1 to 2 pounds per week.

Personal Success: The third component is to focus on the positive aspects of your weight-loss. Try to celebrate small achievements along the way so you can stay motivated towards your long term goal. These personal achievements will help you keep a positive attitude. By writing these successes in your daily journal, you can acknowledge your accomplishments whether they are baby steps or huge leaps of progress.

Visualization: A mental picture is worth a thousand words. In your mind's eye, envision your weight-loss before it happens. Visualize all aspects of the new you from your appearance to your improved health. Remember, if you can see it, chances are very good you can make that healthy visual a reality.

Maintenance: The fifth and final component is maintaining your weight-loss long after you have achieved your goal. Remember to stick with the healthy behaviors, habits, and attitudes that led you to your goal. Keep up the good work, for there is nothing more gratifying than maintaining an ideal weight and a healthy lifestyle!

WRITING FOR WEIGHT-LOSS SUCCESS

Writing in your daily diet journal should be a key factor for your weight-loss program. It will help you stick to your routine, stay focused, and realize your personal goals. This journal will make it easy to keep track of your food and beverage intake, water consumption, and physical activities.

Weight: Your daily weight is an excellent source of feedback. If you do not own a scale, this is the perfect time to buy one. Each morning before eating breakfast, step on the scale and write that number in your daily journal. This is one of the ways you will be able to track your success during your weight-loss program. Try not to be discouraged if your progress is slow or the scale indicates a weight gain. It is normal for your body to fluctuate within a 1-to-2 pound range possibly due to water retention. Stick with your weight-loss plans because you will see success over the course of weeks and months.

Count Your Calories: Each morning, afternoon, and evening write down all the foods you eat including added sauces, condiments, and seasonings. Don't forget your snacks and beverages because every calorie counts. Log the portion size and the corresponding calories for that amount of food. Calculate the calories per meal, and at the end of the day, determine the total calories you have consumed. Compare that number to your daily goal. If you were over your target number, don't penalize yourself. Simply try again tomorrow. This information is vital to your success because it will help you to identify your strengths and weaknesses, discover your eating patterns, and make healthy food selections.

Nutrition Facts: In addition to counting calories, it is important to keep an eye on the nutritional value of your food choices. Read food labels or consult the Nutritional Facts section located in the back of this book to find information on fat, carbohydrates, protein and fiber content. Keep tabs on all of your nutritional totals in your daily journal, as it may indicate future adjustments for food selections.

THINGS YOU SHOULD KNOW
TO LOSE WEIGHT

SUGGESTED DAILY CALORIES FOR WEIGHT MAINTENANCE

Your total daily calories should be based on your age, gender, body type, and level of physical activity. Here are some suggested daily calorie goals for healthy U.S. adults who are maintaining their ideal weight: active men should consume approximately 2,800 calories per day, active women and sedentary men should eat 2,200 calories, and sedentary women and older adults should strive for 1,600 calories. If you are not sure of how many daily calories you should consume, consult your primary care physician for a recommendation.

1,600 CALORIES	2,200 CALORIES	2,800 CALORIES
Sedentary women and older adults should consume approximately 1,600 calories daily.	Most children, teenage girls, active women and sedentary men should consume approximately 2,200 calories daily. Pregnant or breast-feeding women may need to consume more.	Most teenage boys and active men and some very active women should consume approximately 2,800 calories daily.

SUGGESTED DAILY CALORIES FOR WEIGHT-LOSS

The total number of daily calories for a weight-loss plan will depend on the number of pounds you wish to lose. Once you have determined the daily number of calories that you should eat to maintain your weight based on the chart above, you should decrease your total caloric intake by an average of 500 calories per day for a moderate weight-loss. To proceed in a safe and healthy manner, you can eliminate those 500 calories simply by decreasing the amount of sugars, refined carbohydrates, and alcohol in your diet, most of which provide calories with little nutritional value.

RECOMMENDED DAILY AMOUNT FROM EACH FOOD GROUP

The United States Department of Agriculture is known for its Food Guide, which is a nutritional reference for many health groups and dietary plans. The USDA Food Guide separates the foods you should eat into 6 different categories: fruits, vegetables, grains, lean meat and beans, milk, and oils. The suggested amounts below have been developed to help you select the proper amount of food to eat from each group on a daily basis. Each group provides you with a different set of essential nutrients. By following the recommended serving sizes, you can be assured that you are getting the proper amounts of protein, fats, carbohydrates, fiber, vitamins, and minerals. This guide can be adjusted to suit your personal needs.

DAILY AMOUNT OF FOOD FROM EACH GROUP

Calorie Level	1,200	1,400	1,600	1,800	2,000	2,200	2,400	2,600	2,800	3,000
Food Group	Food group amounts shown in cup (C) or ounce (oz), with number of servings (srv) in parentheses. Oils are shown in grams									
Fruits	1 C (2 srv)	1.5 C (3 srv)	1.5 C (3 srv)	1.5 C (3 srv)	2 C (4 srv)	2 C (4 srv)	2 C (4 srv)	2 C (4 srv)	2.5 C (5 srv)	2.5 C (5 srv)
Vegetables	1.5 C (3 srv)	1.5 C (2 srv)	2 C (4 srv)	2.5 C (5 srv)	2.5 C (5 srv)	3 C (6 srv)	3 C (6 srv)	3.5 C (7 srv)	3.5C (7 srv)	4 C (8 srv)
Grains	4 oz	5 oz	5 oz	6 oz	6 oz	7 oz	8 oz	9 oz	10 oz	10 oz
Lean Meat & Beans	3 oz	4 oz	5 oz	5 oz	5.5 oz	6 oz	6.5 oz	6.5 oz	7 oz	7 oz
Milk	2 C	2 C	3 C	3 C	3 C	3 C	3 C	3 C	3 C	3 C
Oils	17 g	17 g	22 g	24 g	27 g	29 g	31 g	34 g	36 g	44 g

HOW MANY SERVINGS SHOULD I EAT?

The USDA Food Guide provides a range of serving sizes within each food group. If you are on a weight-loss plan, try to eat within the number of suggested servings to sustain a healthy metabolism. Remember: to lose weight, you must reduce the number of total calories your body is used to consuming. Therefore, it is extremely important to select foods rich in essential vitamins, minerals and nutrients to feel good and to control your appetite. Within the suggested food groups, consider eating dark green leafy vegetables, whole grain bread, cereal and pasta, lean beef, fish and skinless chicken, and low-fat or fat-free dairy products. Use fats, oils and sweets very sparingly.

A HANDY MEASURING SYSTEM

Many people wonder about portion sizes. It is not always convenient to travel with a food scale or measuring cup. An easier way is to look at your hand. The palm of your hand is the approximate portion size for a 3-ounce piece of chicken, beef, or fish. The size of your thumb is a good estimate for one ounce of cheese. Your clenched fist is about the size of one cup of vegetables. Whether you are eating out or at home, you will always be certain on how much food is a proper portion.

WATER WORKS WONDERS

Drinking 8 eight-ounce glasses of water each day is an excellent addition to your routine. Try drinking a glass before and during each meal to promote feeling full and therefore encouraging the body to eat less. Sometimes an indication of hunger, along with fatigue or headaches, is actually a sign of dehydration. The average adult loses over 2 quarts of water each day. Once your body sends you a message that it is thirsty, you are already dehydrated.

Not only will drinking water at regular intervals keep you hydrated, it can also help you keep your calories down. If you can get used to drinking water at meals instead of a 20 oz. bottle of soda or an alcoholic beverage, you can reduce approximately 250 calories at each meal.

THE NUTRITION FACTS LABEL

Most packaged foods have a nutrition facts label. Use this information to make healthy choices quickly and easily.

Nutrition Facts

Serving Size 1 cup (228g)
Servings Per Container 2

Amount per Serving

Calories 250 Calories from Fat 110

% Daily Value*

Total Fat 12g	**18%**
Saturated Fat 3g	**15%**
Trans Fat 3g	
Cholesterol 30mg	**10%**
Sodium 470mg	**20%**
Total Carbohydrate 31g	**10%**
Dietary Fiber 0g	**0%**
Sugars 5g	
Protein 5g	

Vitamin A	**4%**
Vitamin C	**2%**
Calcium	**20%**
Iron	**4%**

* Percent Daily Values are based on a 2,000 calorie diet. Your Daily Values may be higher or lower depending on your calorie needs.

	Calories:	2,000	2,500
Total Fat	Less than	65g	80g
Sat Fat	Less than	20g	25g
Cholesterol	Less than	300mg	300mg
Sodium	Less than	2,400mg	2,400mg
Total Carbohydrate		300g	375g
Dietary Fiber		25g	30g

LABEL AT A GLANCE

Start Here: Check the serving size and servings per container

Calories: 400 or more calories per serving is considered high. Note the calories from fat.

Daily Values: 5%=low, 20%=high

Limit These Nutrients: Eating too much fat, saturated fat, trans fat, cholesterol, or sodium may put you at an increased health risk for diseases such as heart disease, some cancers, or high blood pressure.

Get Enough of These Nutrients: Most Americans do not receive the proper amount of fiber, vitamins A & C, calcium or iron from their diets. Eating enough of these nutrients can limit your risk of diseases such as osteoporosis and heart disease.

Daily Values Footnote: This footnote makes recommendations for key nutrients based on diets of 2,000 and 2,500 daily calories.

A BREAKDOWN OF THE NUTRITION FACTS LABEL

The first place to look when selecting foods at the market is the product label. Check out **"Nutrition Facts"** for the ingredient list, serving size, calories, amounts, nutrients, portions, and percentage of daily nutritional values. Often you will see "enriched" food sources for wheat or pasta. This is an indication that vitamins or minerals have been added for nutrition. Commonly added nutrients are calcium, thiamin, riboflavin, niacin, iron, and folic acid. The ingredient list tells you exactly what is in the food including nutrients and whether fat or sugar have been added. The ingredients are also listed in descending order by weight.

What Is a Serving Size?: When hunger strikes and a type of food calls out to you, it is important to look at the label for serving size information. The Nutrition Facts label indicates the quantity of food per portion and the number of servings in the package. Serving sizes are now standardized to make it easier to compare foods in familiar units like cups, pieces, grams, or metric amounts. According to the sample label on the previous page, one serving of food equals one cup containing 250 calories. If you ate the whole package, you would have consumed two cups or 500 calories.

All Calories Are Not Created Equal: Calories provide a concrete measure of how much energy you receive from a serving size of a selected food. If you are overweight, chances are you consume more calories than your body needs on a daily basis. You should also be aware of how many calories per serving come from fat. In the sample label, there are 250 calories in a serving, and 110 of those come from fat. That means almost half of the calories are from fat. If you ate two servings or 500 calories, 220 would come from fat, which is 44 percent. To lose weight, select foods with 20 percent or less calories from fat per serving. These can be from proteins, dairy products, and whole grain breads, cereals, and pasta. Most fresh fruits and vegetables are naturally low in fat.

Keep Tabs on Cholesterol: Cholesterol is a fat-like substance present in all animal foods, such as meat, poultry, fish, milk and milk products, and egg yolks. It's a good idea to select lean meats, avoid eating the skin of poultry, and use low-fat milk products. Egg yolks and organ meats, like liver, are high in cholesterol. Plant foods, such as fruit and vegetables, do not contain cholesterol. Why is this important information? Eating foods high in dietary cholesterol increases blood cholesterol in many people, which increases their risk for heart disease. Most health authorities suggest dietary cholesterol should be limited to 300 mg or less per day.

Salt and Sodium: It's important to include some salt in your diet, but it should be limited to 2,400 mg per day. You can keep track of your daily intake by looking at the Nutrition Facts label. Go easy on luncheon and cured meats, cheeses, canned soups and vegetables, and soy sauce. Look for no-salt-added products at your supermarket. Be cautious and avoid adding table salt to your food. Each teaspoon of salt adds 2,000 mg of sodium to your diet. So put down the salt shaker and re-train your taste buds.

Sugar - How Sweet it Isn't: Sugar is an ingredient that is found in almost every food product. If you are counting calories, it is important to look at the list of ingredients to identify all sources of sugar. Obvious foods that add sugar are jams, ice cream, canned fruit and chocolate milk. You will also find it in cereals, sauces, frozen foods, and salad dressings. Here's a list of common sweeteners that are essentially sugar: white sugar, honey, sucrose, fructose, maltose, lactose, syrup, corn syrup, high-fructose corn syrup, molasses, and fruit-juice concentrate. If these terms are found in the first four listings on the label, that food is likely to be very high in sugar. Hint: labels are listed in grams. Consider 4 grams to equal 1 teaspoon of sugar. Total daily intake for all added sugar sources not found naturally in the food itself, should be a maximum 6 teaspoons a day.

Carbohydrates: Breads, cereals, rice, and pasta provide carbohydrates, which are excellent sources of energy. If you are on a weight-loss plan, it is important to include them in your diet because they provide vitamins, minerals, and fiber. One serving of carbohydrates equals one slice of bread, one ounce of ready- to-eat cereal, or 1/2 cup cooked cereal, rice or pasta. Focus on complex carbohydrates, such as whole grain breads, cereals, and brown rice. Keep these foods healthy by not adding additional butter, margarine, cream, cheese, sugar, oils, and fat. Limit refined carbohydrates, such as white flour and sugar, as well as processed foods like pre-packaged candy, cookies, cakes, and chips.

Fruits & Vegetables: Fruits and vegetables can be works of art if you select a rainbow of nine colorful choices throughout your day. For example, eat a yellow banana, green broccoli, orange carrots, a red apple, purple cabbage, and blueberries. Rotate your selections to get the most from your foods. Fruits and vegetables provide vitamins A, C, and folate, and minerals like iron, potassium, and magnesium. Keep in mind that it is important to eat these foods as fresh as possible, preferably raw, and avoid adding butter, mayonnaise, and high-fat salad dressings. When possible, choose the actual piece of fruit, like an apple, over juice.

Protein: The USDA Food Guide suggests eating cooked lean meat as a source of protein for optimum health. Protein provides an essential supply of B vitamins, zinc, and iron. Make sure you get enough of these nutrients by combining a variety of choices, such as lean cuts of beef, pork, veal, lamb, chicken, turkey, fish, and shellfish. Other protein possibilities are eggs, beans, nut butters, tofu, dried nuts, and seeds. Try to choose lean cuts of meat, remove the skin from poultry, trim away all visible fat, go easy on egg yolks, and eat nuts and seeds sparingly.

Fat: As a food source, fat supplies energy and essential fatty acids to your body. Fat-soluble vitamins like A, D, E, K and carotenoids need fat to be absorbed into the body. Not all types of fat are healthy, however, especially saturated fats found in whole milk, butter, ice cream, poultry skin, and palm oil. Unsaturated fats, found mainly in vegetable oils, do not increase blood cholesterol.

A third category called Trans Fat is formed when liquid oils are made into solid fats, like shortening and hard margarine. This type of fat is dangerous because it raises blood cholesterol and increases the risk of coronary heart disease, which is one of the leading causes of death in the United States. Foods high in Trans Fat are processed foods made with partially hydrogenated vegetable oils, such as vegetable shortenings. These oils can be found in crackers, cookies, candies, snack foods, fried foods, and baked goods. It is difficult to avoid all foods with Trans Fat so the ideal goal would be to limit your intake of processed foods as much as possible.

Foods With Healthy Sources of Fat: Try choosing vegetable oils like olive, canola, soybean, sunflower, and corn. Avoid coconut and palm kernel oils. Consider adding fish to your menu twice a week. Salmon and mackerel have omega-3 fatty acids, which offer protection against heart disease. Choose lean meats like skinless chicken, lean beef, and pork. Avoid all fried foods. Watch your fat calories because they contain nine calories per gram, compared to carbohydrates and protein, which have only four calories per gram.

WHAT ARE THE DIFFERENT TYPES OF FAT?

FATS & THEIR SOURCES

SATURATED FATS: Limit these fats. Saturated fats tend to raise blood cholesterol. Foods that contain higher amounts of saturated fats include high fat dairy products (like cheese, whole milk, cream, and regular ice cream), butter, fatty meats, lard, palm oil, and coconut oil.

TRANS FATTY ACIDS: Limit these fats. Foods that are high in trans fatty acids tend to raise blood cholesterol as well. These foods include those high in partially hydrogenated vegetable oils, such as hard margarine and shortenings. Foods with a high amount of this type of fat include some commercially fried foods and some baked goods.

DIETARY CHOLESTEROL: Limit cholesterol. Foods that are high in cholesterol also tend to raise blood cholesterol. These foods include liver and other organ meats, egg yolks, and dairy fat.

UNSATURATED FATS: Unsaturated fats and oils do not raise blood cholesterol. These types of fats occur in vegetable oils such as olive, canola and corn oils, most nuts, avocados, and fatty fish like salmon. Some fish, such as salmon, tuna, and mackerel, contain omega-3 fatty acids that may offer protection against heart disease. This is the best type of fat to include in your diet, just be sure to take care to avoid excess calories.

BEST SOURCES FOR ESSENTIAL NUTRIENTS

BEST SOURCES FOR CALCIUM

Milk & dairy	yogurt, cheese, milk
Seafood	sardines, pink salmon, perch, blue crab, clams
Various vegetables	collard, turnip, dandelion greens, spinach
Peas/beans/legumes	soybeans/tofu, cowpeas, white beans
Fortified foods	cereals, soy milk, oatmeal

BEST SOURCES FOR IRON

Shellfish	clams, oysters, shrimp
Organ meats	liver, giblets
Beans/legumes/peas	soy, white, kidney, lima, navy, lentils
Lean meats	beef, duck, lamb
Various fruit/vegetables	spinach, prune juice, tomato puree/paste

BEST SOURCES FOR VITAMIN A, C, E & POTASSIUM

SOURCES OF VITAMIN A:

Organ meats	liver, giblets
Dark leafy vegetables	collard, turnip, mustard greens, kale
Orange fruit/vegetables	carrots, sweet potato, pumpkin, squash

SOURCES OF VITAMIN C:

Various fruits	guava, kiwi, orange, grapefruit, strawberries, cantaloupe, papaya, pineapple, mango
Various vegetables	red/green sweet pepper, brussel sprouts, broccoli, sweet potato, cauliflower, kale

SOURCES OF VITAMIN E:

Fortified foods	ready-to-eat cereals
Seeds & nuts	sunflower seeds, almonds, hazelnuts, pine nuts
Oils	sunflower, cottonseed, safflower, canola, peanut

SOURCES OF POTASSIUM:

Various vegetables	sweet potato, tomato puree/paste, beet greens, potato, carrot juice, winter squash, spinach
Beans/legumes/peas	white beans, soybeans, lentils, kidney beans
Milk & dairy	yogurt, milk
Various fruits	prune juice, bananas, peaches, prunes, apricots

DIETARY GUIDELINES FOR AMERICANS

INCLUDING VARIOUS FOODS IN YOUR DIET will allow your body to receive the energy (calories), protein, vitamins, minerals, and fiber you need to maintain proper health.

COMBINE A HEALTHY DIET WITH PHYSICAL ACTIVITY to improve your weight or maintain your weight. Maintaining a healthy weight reduces the risk of related diseases, such as high blood pressure, heart disease, a stroke, certain cancers, and the most common kind of diabetes.

CHOOSE A DIET LOW IN FAT, SATURATED FAT AND CHOLESTEROL to reduce your risk of heart disease and certain types of cancer. Because fat contains more than twice the calories of an equal amount of carbohydrates or protein, a diet low in fat can help you maintain a healthy weight.

INCLUDE PLENTY OF VEGETABLES, FRUITS, AND WHOLE GRAIN products in your diet. These foods provide essential vitamins, minerals, fiber, and complex carbohydrates. They are also generally lower in fat.

USE SUGARS ONLY IN MODERATION. A diet with high amounts of sugars has unnecessary calories and too few nutrients for the majority of adults. Excess sugar can also contribute to tooth decay.

USE SALT AND OTHER FORMS OF SODIUM IN MODERATION to help reduce your risk of high blood pressure.

IF YOU DRINK ALCOHOLIC BEVERAGES, DO SO IN MODERATION. Alcoholic beverages supply calories, but little or no nutrients. Drinking alcohol is also the cause of many health problems and accidents and can lead to addiction.

EXERCISE FOR FITNESS AND FUN

The previous sections discussed the importance of consuming fewer calories, eating less fat, and redefining your food choices. This knowledge will help you shed unwanted pounds. Now, try including exercise to your weight loss program so you accelerate the number of calories your body burns.

An additional key element for success is developing an exercise program. Choose activities that can be done each day so you can incorporate them into your daily routine. The length of time it takes to change from a sedentary to an active lifestyle can range from three weeks to three months. Get started by creating simple habits like taking the stairs and walking more often. Slowly add more exercises and increase the intensity as your body adjusts to each new activity.

So what is the best exercise regiment for you to embark on? The answer depends on your personality, interests, and individual abilities. The optimal solution is to choose an exercise program you will enjoy doing, and one that you will look forward to each day.

You have a wide range of options when creating a fitness plan. It can be slow, moderate, or physically challenging. You can do it all at one time, or integrate it into two or three segments over the course of your day. So build a physical activity plan that fits into your daily calendar, and keep in mind the common ingredient for any successful exercise program is to bring a measure of pleasure into it.

In addition to having fun and feeling energized, physical activity provides added perks, such as building muscle tone, curbing your appetite, and increasing your metabolism. One by-product built into a fitness-oriented lifestyle is improved overall health. It has been found that regular physical exercise reduces the risks of cancer, cardiovascular disease, and diabetes. It also provides psychological benefits, such as increased self-esteem and feelings of confidence. Taking action toward physical fitness will make you look great and feel like a winner.

A COMPLETE PHYSICAL FITNESS PROGRAM

Your mission is to burn calories. Your new fitness program should include three essential elements for successful, long-term weight-loss and maintenance: the first element is to include aerobic activities, which provide cardiovascular benefits; the second element is a resistance or strength training program for improving muscle tone; and the third element is to consider integrating a basic stretching routine into your daily schedule to develop flexibility.

Before embarking on your mission, see a doctor to obtain a health clearance if you have unique health issues, injuries, or physical limitations. When you are ready to exercise, warm up slowly and be gentle on your body. It's the only one you've got, so take care of it as you work your way into top physical form.

Aerobic Activities: An aerobic activity is any type of body movement that speeds up your heart rate and breathing. It improves your ability to utilize oxygen, which increases your cardiovascular health. You can participate in aerobic activities almost anywhere: step classes at a gym, running in a park or on a stationary bicycle in your home environment. The minimum amount of time for adult daily exercise is 30 minutes, and children benefit from 60 minutes per day. Keep in mind these numbers are a general estimate and should be tailored to fit individual needs. In all cases, use common sense when exercising and be sure to listen to your body. A general guideline for physical activity is to safely challenge your body while gradually stretching your limits.

Resistance & Strength Training: Once you have a personalized aerobic program that fits your style, consider adding a crucial piece of the puzzle to your fitness regime. Resistance and strength training will firm up muscles as the unwanted pounds melt away. This type of exercise should be done for 20 to 30 minutes, three times a week. It includes lifting hand-held weights, using machines at a gym, or working out with videos in your home. If you choose to go to the gym, consult with professionals and learn how to correctly use the equipment.

Stretching & Flexibility: Stretching and flexibility are often neglected components of physical activity. Preparing the body for movement, and keeping it injury-free, should be built into every fitness program. Stretching and flexibility training is designed to develop range of motion, increase muscle elasticity, and achieve muscle balance. Stretching can also speed up recovery in preparation for the next fitness session. You should never stretch your body when it's cold or stiff. Be sure to start your physical activity with 10 to 15 minutes of slow movement until your muscles have warmed up. Mild stretching can be done at a mid-point in your daily training and again at the completion of the exercise program.

The best type of overall stretching routine is one that starts with the head and neck, working down towards the toes. It uses slow stretches that are held for a minimum of 10 seconds each. Avoid quick-pulling motions that put stress on muscles and joints. Choose abdominal exercises that support the lower back region. In all cases, consult with a professional for advice before beginning a strength and flexibility program.

INCORPORATE ACTIVITIES INTO YOUR DAILY ROUTINE

If you are not the type of person who enjoys going to a gym, consider making your home environment a personalized recreational center. All forms of physical activity burn calories. So let's look at your daily chores in a new light: vacuuming for one hour burns 220 calories, grocery shopping requires 180 calories, and raking leaves expends 90 calories. If you have access to stairs, perhaps you might use them as your personal stair-stepper. Walking up stairs in an easy and moderate manner for 15 minutes burns 120 calories.

Enjoy being outdoors? Try an afternoon of gardening, sweeping, raking leaves or mowing the lawn to tone up your arms, legs, and abdominals while you whittle away an additional 270 calories per hour. If you live in an area where it snows, you have hit the jackpot as shoveling snow consumes almost 600 calories per hour. Combining a few of these forms of aerobic activity is the equivalent of spending a couple of hours in the gym.

WALKING

Perhaps home maintenance is not your idea of enjoyable exercise. Take a closer look at good old-fashioned walking. On a nice day, consider a stroll around your neighborhood. In cold or rainy weather, go to a local indoor mall and log miles while you glance at shoppers and window displays. This is a cost-effective activity that simply requires a good pair of walking shoes.

Walking may sound too good to be true, but it is an aerobic activity that burns calories. Consider the fact that walking at 2 mph, which is approximately a 30-minute mile, burns 200 calories. Walking a 20-minute mile at a 3 mph pace uses 240 calories. Walking a moderate, 15-minute mile, for an average of 4 mph, burns 300 calories. The faster you walk the more calories you will burn.

Measuring a Mile: You may wonder how far you should walk to log one mile. After all, there are no standards when it comes to the length of suburban streets. Here are a few methods of calculating distance. You can use a car to drive your neighborhood streets and look at your odometer to calculate mileage, or your may purchase a small pedometer to count your steps. The U.S. Surgeon General has recommended walking 30 minutes daily to strive toward a weekly goal of 10,000 steps, or roughly 5 miles. Those on a weight-loss program should strive for a minimum of 12,000 to 15,000 steps, which should take about 45 minutes per day.

HEALTH BENEFITS OF PHYSICAL ACTIVITY

Still need convincing that it is essential to change from a sedentary lifestyle to one that includes daily physical activity? Here are a few facts that might influence your decision: it has been found that regular physical activity reduces the risk of dying prematurely; exercise reduces the risk of developing heart disease, cancer, diabetes, and high blood pressure, and promotes psychological well being. Exercise also helps decrease or eliminate depression and anxiety. Participating in physical activities is also an effective way to lose weight and maintain weight-loss.

EXERCISE AND WEIGHT CONTROL

Carrying around too much body fat is a nuisance. Many people fight the "battle of the bulge" through diet alone because exercise is not always convenient. Few of today's occupations require physical activity and many people spend hours behind desks and computers. In addition, much of our leisure time is spent in sedentary pursuits. To reverse this trend, it is important to adjust your attitude and find time to exercise each day. Here's a look at the most common reasons people use to avoid physical activity:

1. I don't have the time.
2. I'm too tired and I don't feel like it.
3. I'm not very good at exercising.
4. It's not convenient to get to my workout place.
5. I'm afraid and embarrassed.

Overweight or Overfat?: Being overweight and overfat are two different dilemmas. Some people, such as athletes, have a muscular physique and weigh more than average for their age and height, but their body composition, which is the amount of fat versus lean body mass (muscle, bone, organs and tissue), is within an acceptable range. Others can weigh within the range of U.S. guidelines, yet can carry around too much fat. Use exercise as a way to balance your body fat percentage. An easy self-test is to pinch the thickness of fat at your waist and abdomen. If you can pinch more than an inch of fat, excluding muscles, chances are you have too much body fat.

Energy Balance and Counting Calories: Losing weight boils down to a simple mathematical formula: consume fewer calories than you burn. Learn how to balance energy intake (food) with energy output (calories burned by physical activity). If you take in more calories than your body needs to perform your day's activities, it will be stored as fat. Therefore, the only solution is to consume the proper amount of calories that your body needs to maintain good health. Then exercise so your body can utilize the stored fat. The end result will be your desired weight-loss.

CALORIES BURNED FOR TYPICAL PHYSICAL ACTIVITIES

LIGHT ACTIVITIES - 150 or less	CAL/HR.
Billiards	140
Lying down/sleeping	60
Office work	140
Sitting	80
Standing	100

MODERATE ACTIVITIES - 150-350	CAL/HR.
Aerobic Dancing	340
Ballroom dancing	210
Bicycling (5 mph)	170
Bowling	160
Canoeing (2.5 mph)	170
Dancing (social)	210
Gardening (moderate)	270
Golf (with cart)	180
Golf (without cart)	320
Grocery shopping	180
Horseback riding (sitting trot)	250
Light housework/cleaning, etc.	250
Ping pong	270
Swimming (20 yards/min)	290
Tennis (recreational doubles)	310
Vacuuming	220
Volleyball (recreational)	260
Walking (2 mph)	200
Walking (3 mph)	240
Walking (4 mph)	300

CALORIES BURNED FOR TYPICAL PHYSICAL ACTIVITIES

VIGOROUS ACTIVITIES - 350 or MORE	CAL/HR.
Aerobics (step)	440
Backpacking (10 lb load)	540
Badminton	450
Basketball (competitive)	660
Basketball (leisure)	390
Bicycling (10 mph)	375
Bicycling (13 mph)	600
Cross country skiing (leisurely)	460
Cross country skiing (moderate)	660
Hiking	460
Ice skating (9 mph)	384
Jogging (5 mph)	550
Jogging (6 mph)	690
Racquetball	620
Rollerblading	384
Rowing machine	540
Running (8 mph)	900
Scuba diving	570
Shoveling snow	580
Soccer	580
Spinning	650
Stair climber machine	480
Swimming (50 yards/min.)	680
Water aerobics	400
Water skiing	480
Weight training (30 sec. b/w sets)	760
Weight training (60 sec. b/w sets)	570

NOTES

YOUR PERSONAL PROFILE

Begin your weight-loss program by completing some helpful information so you can assess your current physical state, habits, and eating patterns. This information will assist you in identifying the areas of your diet and health that need improvement.

Start out by completing statistics regarding your age, weight, height, body fat percentage, and Body Mass Index (see page 14). If you are a member of a gym, you can set up an appointment to get your body fat measured for a small fee. There are also scales available that will calculate your body fat percentage. Another option is purchasing an at home body fat analyzer, which is small hand-held device that measures your fat. These analyzers are affordable and can be purchased online or at your local health and fitness retailer.

Visit your primary care physician to find out important information regarding your health. Have your doctor measure your cholesterol, triglycerides, blood pressure and glucose levels. You can also check with your local drug store and see if the pharmacy offers this service for a nominal fee. This information will help you determine if you are at risk for certain diseases or conditions. In addition, these levels will also factor into the food choices you make when creating your diet. For example, if you have high blood pressure, you may want to reduce your sodium intake. Therefore, you should try to avoid foods with added salt. High levels of cholesterol and triglycerides (over 160 mg/dL for cholesterol, over 200 mg/dL for triglycerides) can put you at risk for heart related diseases. In this instance, you should limit the amount of saturated fats, trans fats and dietary cholesterol found in high fat dairy and meat products.

Finally, assess your current eating and physical habits. Document the types of foods you currently eat, when you typically have meals, and any other dietary requirements that you have. If you are active, write down the exercises you participate in and how often you do them. You can also answer some additional questions to help you define problem areas and assist you in determining the weight-loss plan that is most beneficial for your needs.

YOUR PERSONAL PROFILE

Complete the following personal health profile. You can request necessary information from your primary health care provider.

YOUR PROFILE

Name: _____   Total Cholesterol: _____

Age: _____   Triglycerides: _____

Weight: _____   HDL Cholesterol:_____

Height: _____   LDL Cholesterol: _____

Body Fat Percentage: _____   Blood Pressure:_____

Body Mass Index*: _____   Glucose: _____

*Refer to page 14 to determine your BMI

Current Diet & Eating Habits: (vegetarian, low carb, snack often, compulsive eating, etc.)

_____

_____

_____

_____

_____

Current Physical Activity: (sedentary, moderately active, very active) _____

_____

_____

_____

_____

Other Current Habits: (smoking, drinking, lack of sleep, etc.)_____

_____

_____

_____

_____

The following questions will assist you in developing your weight-loss program. When choosing a specific diet program, determining your strengths and weaknesses will help you figure out what plan is right for you.

QUESTIONS TO ASK

Which best describes your daily eating habits?

❑ 3 average meals
❑ Graze frequently
❑ One large meal/little else

What types of food do you crave the most?

❑ Meat/fish
❑ Fruit/vegetables
❑ Bread/cereals/rice
❑ Sweets

Do you typically eat out or prepare food for yourself?

❑ I usually cook my own food
❑ I eat out or have pre-made meals

What is your weight-loss goal?

❑ Lose 20 or more pounds
❑ Maintain weight
❑ Lose a little weight
❑ Improve health

What is your fitness goal?

❑ Decrease fat
❑ Gain muscle
❑ Improve strength

Describe your body type:

❑ Overweight
❑ Average
❑ Muscular

What length of plan would you want to consider?

❑ Less than 1 month
❑ 1-3 months
❑ 3-6 months
❑ 6 or more months

What particular event do you want to lose weight for (if any)?

_____

_____

_____

_____

When developing your weight-loss program and goals, be sure to take into account the answers that you have noted above. These answers will factor into your decision when choosing the program that would be most effective and best suit your needs.

YOUR PERSONAL WEIGHT-LOSS
GOALS, PLANS, & ACHIEVEMENTS

Once you have created a weight-loss goal and selected a program, write down the specific information in this section. This way, you can easily keep track of the daily requirements for your program. Begin by writing down the name of your weight-loss plan. Be sure to determine your time frame for the program, including the start and end date. Use the space provided to describe your personal goal and the diet plan that you will be using.

You can further outline your diet by recording the specific number of daily calories your plan allows. You can also fill in the total grams of fat, protein, carbohydrates, fiber, and ounces of water that you should consume. Documenting this information will assist you when making your daily food choices and help you to stay within your total daily calorie allotment. You will easily be able to keep track of these totals when you calculate your nutritional totals using the daily diet journal pages.

Decide if you want to incorporate an exercise plan into your weight-loss program. If so, you can outline the activities that you would like to include in this section and schedule them into your routine.

Since you are now on your way to losing weight and looking better, you can also look forward to documenting your results. In the space indicated, write down your current measurements and your desired measurements. Once you have completed your program, you can fill in your final information and compare your end results to your original statistics.

Additionally, you can post a "before" and "after" photo so you can visually compare your body from the start of the program to the end. This is a very satisfying way to assess your results.

Several sets of pages have been supplied so you can create up to three different plans. If you begin one plan and find that it does not work for you, use the additional pages to outline a new goal and plan, and include the adjustments that you need to make.

Complete the following information based on your desired goal & plan:

NAME OF PLAN: _____   START DATE: 1-19-08

LENGTH OF PLAN: _____   END DATE: _____

1.) DESCRIPTION OF GOAL

5'8" 80

22 BMI

2.) DESCRIPTION OF DIET PLAN

Depending on the amount of calories allotted daily per your diet, list below
the daily targets that you would like to meet each day:

TOTAL DAILY CALORIES: _____

     Fat grams: _____   Carb grams: _____

     Protein grams: _____   Fiber grams: _____

     Water (oz.): _____   Other: _____

3.) DESCRIPTION OF EXERCISE PLAN

Treadmill 2x daily

weights 3x week

If you are also including a fitness program into your plan, you can outline
the activities that you would like to accomplish for each day of the week:

Mon: _____   Thurs: _____

Tues: _____   Fri: _____

Wed: _____   Sat/Sun: _____

After you have completed your desired program, complete the following information so you can review your results!

1-19-08

4.) RESULTS

STATISTICS	BEFORE	DESIRED	AFTER
Weight	197.2		
Body Fat %			
Body Mass Index	30%		
Chest	41		
Waist	37		
Hips	46½		
Thigh	26		
Bicep			

BEFORE AND AFTER PHOTOS:

Be proud of your results! Take a "before" and "after" photo and paste them here so you can compare and track your progress:

YOUR PERSONAL GOALS, PLANS, & ACHIEVEMENTS

Complete the following information based on your desired goal & plan:

NAME OF PLAN: _____   START DATE: _____

LENGTH OF PLAN: _____   END DATE: _____

1.) DESCRIPTION OF GOAL

_____

_____

_____

2.) DESCRIPTION OF DIET PLAN

_____

_____

_____

Depending on the amount of calories allotted daily per your diet, list below the daily targets that you would like to meet each day:

TOTAL DAILY CALORIES: _____

Fat gms: _____   Carb gms: _____

Protein gms: _____   Fiber gms: _____

Water/oz.: _____   Other: _____

3.) DESCRIPTION OF EXERCISE PLAN

_____

_____

_____

If you are also including a fitness program into your plan, you can outline the activities that you would like to accomplish for each day of the week.

Mon: _____   Thurs: _____

Tues: _____   Fri: _____

Wed: _____   Sat/Sun: _____

After you have completed your desired program, complete the following information so you can review your results!

4.) RESULTS

STATISTICS	BEFORE	DESIRED	AFTER
Weight			
Body Fat %			
Body Mass Index			
Chest			
Waist			
Hips			
Thigh			
Bicep			

BEFORE AND AFTER PHOTOS:

Be proud of your results! Take a "before" and "after photo and paste them here so you can compare and track your progress.

place
"BEFORE"
photo
here

place
"AFTER"
photo
here

YOUR PERSONAL GOALS, PLANS, & ACHIEVEMENTS

Complete the following information based on your desired goal & plan:

NAME OF PLAN: _____   START DATE: _____

LENGTH OF PLAN: _____   END DATE: _____

1.) DESCRIPTION OF GOAL

_____

_____

_____

2.) DESCRIPTION OF DIET PLAN

_____

_____

_____

Depending on the amount of calories allotted daily per your diet, list below the daily targets that you would like to meet each day:

TOTAL DAILY CALORIES: _____

Fat grams:_____   Carb grams: _____

Protein grams: _____   Fiber grams:_____

Water (oz.): _____   Other: _____

3.) DESCRIPTION OF EXERCISE PLAN

_____

_____

_____

If you are also including a fitness program into your plan, you can outline the activities that you would like to accomplish for each day of the week.

Mon:_____   Thurs:_____

Tues:_____   Fri: _____

Wed: _____   Sat/Sun: _____

After you have completed your desired program, complete the following information so you can review your results!

4.) RESULTS

STATISTICS	BEFORE	DESIRED	AFTER
Weight			
Body Fat %			
Body Mass Index			
Chest			
Waist			
Hips			
Thigh			
Bicep			

BEFORE AND AFTER PHOTOS:

Be proud of your results! Take a "before" and "after" photo and paste them here so you can compare and track your progress:

NOTES

THE SECRET TO WEIGHT-LOSS:

KEEPING TRACK OF

WHAT YOU EAT

For human weight, one pound of fat is equal to 3,500 stored calories. If weight-loss is viewed in the most simplistic of terms, it can be determined as the amount of calories consumed versus the amount of calories burned. If you burn more calories than you eat, then ideally you should lose weight.

The most important aspect of weight-loss is to be aware of how much food and the total number of calories you consume on a daily basis. This awareness can be created through the use of this diet journal. Why is it important to keep track of what you eat? By actively documenting the foods and beverages you consume on a daily basis, you are establishing the following criteria that will help you lose-weight.

Awareness: Keeping a diet journal builds your daily food awareness. Instead of mindlessly consuming meals, this diet journal will help you become conscious of what you are eating, how much, and how often. This awareness will help you realize that maybe you don't need as much food as you are currently eating. Perhaps you can be perfectly satisfied with less. With the use of this journal, you can discover how foods can affect your body. Do you feel sluggish after eating too many fatty foods? Do you feel energetic and refreshed after eating a salad and lean protein? You will also learn what foods have more calories, fat and nutrients than others. If you are aware of what your body needs to lose weight, you can make better, more informed food choices.

Reality: Many dieters do not realize how many calories are included in the foods that they consume. This diet journal allows you to break down your meals into total calories. At the end of each day, you can add up your daily totals. Then you can check and see if you have stayed within the range of calories suggested for your diet. For example, if you have a turkey and swiss bagel with mayo, a bag of chips, a chocolate chip cookie, and a soda for lunch, the calories versus a turkey pita with veggies, popcorn, and yogurt would be twice as much. See the following page for the caloric values for both meals.

TURKEY SWISS BAGEL LUNCH		TURKEY PITA LUNCH	
370	large gourmet deli bagel	170	whole wheat pita
90	3 slices of 1 oz. turkey breast	90	3 slices of 1 oz. turkey breast
220	2 1 oz. slices of swiss cheese	25	1 tbsp grated parmesan cheese
100	1 tbsp mayo	5	1 tsp mustard
275	deli chocolate chip cookie	20	veggies
150	1 oz. snack bag chips	60	2 cups light microwave popcorn
150	12 oz. can soda	120	6 oz. non-fat flavored yogurt
		0	water with lemon

1,355 TOTAL CALORIES (approx.)   490 TOTAL CALORIES (approx.)

Once you realize where the majority of calories are coming from, you can make healthier, low calorie changes and eliminate the excess foods that do not have significant nutritional value. Some foods just have more calories than others. When you realize that an average blueberry scone from your local coffee shop has 450 calories and 17 grams of fat, you may want to choose an alternate breakfast of a whole wheat english muffin, an omelet with 2 egg whites, a 1 oz. slice of ham, tomatoes, onions, bell peppers and a medium banana for 340 calories and 6 grams of fat.

Accountability: Keeping a diet journal forces individuals to account for all food and beverages consumed on a daily basis. Many individuals who are seeking to lose weight allow hidden calories to sneak into their diet. By writing down all of the foods you eat and calculating the daily calorie and nutritional value for all your meals, you are forced to consider how an extra serving of pasta or a dessert will factor into your diet. Many people do not take into consideration their beverages when on a weight-loss program. If you favor whole milk lattés, smoothies, soda, alcoholic drinks, and juices, it is possible to drink as many calories as you get from your food. Be sure to include calories from all beverages, as well as solid food, and then determine whether or not you need to cut back.

Routine: When you start a diet journal, you establish a routine. This routine helps you to maintain a stable, steady progress towards your weight-loss goal. If you have a plan that you can count on for every day of the week, you are more likely to keep with your diet and avoid situations that can sabotage your diet. Even if you end up eating an additional slice of pizza with friends or have a decadent meal with drinks and dessert, you have the benefit of having a solid foundation to which you can return the next day.

HOW TO START

Start out each day by assigning a two-page spread for the current date. Invest in a weight scale so you can accurately measure your weight-loss progress. Since your aim is to lose weight, this is an essential tool for your program. Weigh yourself unclothed when you wake up in the morning, before breakfast, so you can get a fresh reading for the day. Write down this number at the top of the page. Gradually, as you make your progress, you will see this number move closer to your goal. Do not worry if during your program, this number fluctuates up or down. There are many factors, such as water and muscle gain, that can affect your weight. A typical fluctuation can range from 2-3 pounds. Don't let this thwart your program; instead, focus more on your weekly and monthly progress.

Daily Nutritional Intake: Begin by writing down all of the foods that you eat on a daily basis. The daily nutritional intake section is separated into 3 meals: breakfast, lunch, and dinner, as well as a fourth section for snacks. Write down the time you consume each meal, as well as all the items in your meal, including dressing, condiments, and beverages. To accurately assess your daily totals, it is extremely important to include all the items and the quantity of each.

Each meal has a section for comments. You can jot helpful information in this space that will assist you in planning or calculating your daily menu. For example, if you know you are going out to lunch at a restaurant, jot down several healthy menu options that would work with your diet plan.

Calories and Nutritional Values: For each meal, calculate your nutritional totals for calories, fat, carbohydrates, protein, and fiber. You can find the values for the most popular food items in the nutritional information section located in the back of this journal. This type of information can also be found online, or you can purchase a calorie counting book at your local bookstore. There are some books that also cover restaurants and fast food items. In addition, you can refer to the nutrition facts label printed on the container of most pre-packaged foods. Once you have made all of your documentation for the day, use the Daily Totals section to calculate the total number of calories you have consumed. Compare your totals to the number of calories suggested for your program. If you are at your target or under, you are on the right track. If you are a little over, do not worry. Just make some adjustments to your diet and try to choose more low-calorie options. Do your best to avoid diet pitfalls, such as sugar, extra fat, and alcohol.

Exercise and Fitness: This section will encourage you to participate in physical activities on a daily basis. All types of physical activities burn calories so be sure to write down your exercise routine, the length of the session, and the approximate calories utilized by your body. This information can help you recognize your behaviors or habits that may lead to a successful weight-loss journey. It is also a source of reference to help you maintain your ideal body weight in the future.

Weight-loss is determined by the amount of calories consumed versus the amount burned. If you happen to have a "bad eating" day, you can try to make up for the excess calories by adding an additional exercise routine the following day. Since you will be completing this section on a daily basis, motivate yourself by incorporating the activities that you enjoy the most.

Energy Levels: Determine the relationship that your body has with food. Take notice of how your body responds to your weight-loss program. Document your daily overall energy levels at the top of the second page. See how your energy correlates to the types of foods you have included in your program. If you notice that a little extra protein helps you get through your workout, incorporate lean meats in your diet. As you discover these relationships, make adjustments as needed to help you feel your best.

Water Intake: Strive for a total of 8 eight-ounce glasses of water per day. Write down your daily intake to reach your healthy hydration goals. Many times people believe that they are hungry when they are actually thirsty. If you drink water on a normal basis throughout the day, you can maintain a constant level of hydration.

Vitamins and Supplements: This section is a great daily reminder if you are incorporating additional nutrients into your diet program. If you are restricting your daily caloric intake, it can be a good idea to take vitamins and supplements. If you choose to do so, mark it in your journal and be sure to keep track on a daily basis. You can also assess the effectiveness of your supplements over time by comparing your energy levels to the vitamins that you have taken. Also, if you make changes to food that you eat while on your diet, you may want to consider adapting your supplements as well. When in doubt about specific vitamin recommendations, consult with health care professionals.

Daily Servings Guide: Check off your daily food servings in the 6 categories suggested by the Food Guide. Keeping track of this information will allow you to see what food groups you may be consuming too much of and what groups you may not be getting enough from. This can also help you from going over your total number of calories since it breaks down the foods you eat into different limits.

Daily Assessment & Notes: This section will help you observe obstacles and solutions throughout this diet journey. Record your thoughts and feelings as you gradually achieve your weight-loss goals. Stay motivated by recording positive results and reflecting on your progress.

Daily Goals Achieved: This is a quick way to track your daily progress towards your goal. If for any reason you did not meet your daily goal, reflect on the factors that kept you from your goal and write them down in the assessments section. You can then decide on any changes that you can make to your diet or fitness plan to help you stay on track. Incorporate these improvements into your following day.

Daily Nutritional Intake

FOOD AND BEVERAGES

MORNING TIME:	amt.	cal.	fat gms	protein gms	carbs. gms	fiber gms
Tea w/ Sugar						
Cottage Cheese / Pineapple						
BREAKFAST TOTALS						

COMMENTS:

AFTERNOON TIME:	amt.	cal.	fat gms	protein gms	carbs. gms	fiber gms
LUNCH TOTALS						

COMMENTS:

EVENING TIME:	amt.	cal.	fat gms	protein gms	carbs. gms	fiber gms
DINNER TOTALS						

COMMENTS:

☐ low ☐ med ☐ high

ENERGY LEVELS

Daily Nutritional Intake

FOOD AND BEVERAGES

**DAILY GOALS
ACHIEVED**

DAILY TOTALS

SNACKS TIME:		amt.	cal.	fat gms	protein gms	carbs. gms	fiber gms
SNACK TOTALS							

COMMENTS:

_____ Calories

_____ Fat

_____ Protein

_____ Carbohydrates

_____ Fiber

_____ Other

Exercise and Fitness

DAILY PHYSICAL ACTIVITIES

**VITAMINS &
SUPPLEMENTS**

ACTIVITY/ EXERCISE		hrs./ mins.	reps./ sets	------INTENSITY------ low	med	high	cal. burned
TOTAL CALORIES BURNED							

COMMENTS:

Type:
Qty:
Type:
Qty:
Type:
Qty:
Type:
Qty:
Type:
Qty:
Type:
Qty:

Daily Assessment and Notes

OBSTACLES, SOLUTIONS AND THOUGHTS ON YOUR PROGRESS

_____

_____

_____

_____

_____

Helpful Tips
for Effective
Weight-Loss

Try not to eat while
watching television,
driving, reading or
any other activity.
It can make you
lose track of what
and how much you
are eating.

Daily Nutritional Intake

FOOD AND BEVERAGES

MORNING TIME:	amt.	cal.	fat gms	protein gms	carbs. gms	fiber gms
BREAKFAST TOTALS						

COMMENTS:

AFTERNOON TIME:	amt.	cal.	fat gms	protein gms	carbs. gms	fiber gms
LUNCH TOTALS						

COMMENTS:

EVENING TIME:	amt.	cal.	fat gms	protein gms	carbs. gms	fiber gms
DINNER TOTALS						

COMMENTS:

Daily Serving Intake

_____ Fruits
# of servings

_____ Vegetables
# of servings

_____ Grains
# of servings

_____ Meat & Beans
# of servings

_____ Milk & Dairy
# of servings

_____ Oils & Sweets
# of servings

Water Intake

oz.

Daily Nutritional Intake

FOOD AND BEVERAGES

DAILY GOALS
ACHIEVED

DAILY TOTALS

SNACKS TIME:	amt.	cal.	fat gms	protein gms	carbs. gms	fiber gms
SNACK TOTALS						

COMMENTS:

Calories

Fat

Protein

Carbohydrates

Fiber

Other

Exercise and Fitness

DAILY PHYSICAL ACTIVITIES

ACTIVITY/ EXERCISE	hrs./ mins.	reps./ sets	low	med	high	cal. burned
TOTAL CALORIES BURNED						

INTENSITY (spanning low, med, high columns)

COMMENTS:

VITAMINS &
SUPPLEMENTS

Type:
Qty:
Type:
Qty:
Type:
Qty:
Type:
Qty:
Type:
Qty:
Type:
Qty:
Type:
Qty:

Daily Assessment and Notes

OBSTACLES, SOLUTIONS AND THOUGHTS ON YOUR PROGRESS

WEIGHT

Daily Nutritional Intake

FOOD AND BEVERAGES

Celebrate your
success every day.
Be proud of what
you have accom-
plished and contin-
ue to envision the
future you.

MORNING TIME:	amt.	cal.	fat gms	protein gms	carbs. gms	fiber gms
BREAKFAST TOTALS						

COMMENTS:

AFTERNOON TIME:	amt.	cal.	fat gms	protein gms	carbs. gms	fiber gms
LUNCH TOTALS						

COMMENTS:

Daily Serving Intake

_____ Fruits
# of servings

_____ Vegetables
# of servings

_____ Grains
# of servings

_____ Meat & Beans
# of servings

_____ Milk & Dairy
# of servings

_____ Oils & Sweets
# of servings

Water Intake

oz.

EVENING TIME:	amt.	cal.	fat gms	protein gms	carbs. gms	fiber gms
DINNER TOTALS						

COMMENTS:

ENERGY LEVELS

Daily Nutritional Intake

FOOD AND BEVERAGES

DAILY GOALS
ACHIEVED

SNACKS TIME:	amt.	cal.	fat gms	protein gms	carbs. gms	fiber gms
SNACK TOTALS						

COMMENTS:

DAILY TOTALS

Calories

Fat

Protein

Carbohydrates

Fiber

Other

Exercise and Fitness

DAILY PHYSICAL ACTIVITIES

ACTIVITY/ EXERCISE	hrs./ mins.	reps./ sets	INTENSITY low	med	high	cal. burned
TOTAL CALORIES BURNED						

COMMENTS:

VITAMINS &
SUPPLEMENTS

Type:
Qty:
Type:
Qty:
Type:
Qty:
Type:
Qty:
Type:
Qty:
Type:
Qty:

Daily Assessment and Notes

OBSTACLES, SOLUTIONS AND THOUGHTS ON YOUR PROGRESS

Daily Nutritional Intake

FOOD AND BEVERAGES

Adding new food
and variety to your
plan will help keep
your diet interest-
ing and keep you
motivated.

MORNING TIME:	amt.	cal.	fat gms	protein gms	carbs. gms	fiber gms
BREAKFAST TOTALS						

COMMENTS:

AFTERNOON TIME:	amt.	cal.	fat gms	protein gms	carbs. gms	fiber gms
LUNCH TOTALS						

COMMENTS:

Daily Serving Intake

____ Fruits
# of servings

____ Vegetables
# of servings

____ Grains
# of servings

____ Meat & Beans
# of servings

____ Milk & Dairy
# of servings

____ Oils & Sweets
# of servings

EVENING TIME:	amt.	cal.	fat gms	protein gms	carbs. gms	fiber gms
DINNER TOTALS						

Water Intake

oz. _____

COMMENTS:

Daily Nutritional Intake

FOOD AND BEVERAGES

DAILY GOALS
ACHIEVED

DAILY TOTALS

SNACKS TIME:	amt.	cal.	fat gms	protein gms	carbs. gms	fiber gms
SNACK TOTALS						

COMMENTS:

Calories

Fat

Protein

Carbohydrates

Fiber

Other

Exercise and Fitness

DAILY PHYSICAL ACTIVITIES

VITAMINS &
SUPPLEMENTS

ACTIVITY/ EXERCISE	hrs./ mins.	reps./ sets	------INTENSITY------			cal. burned
			low	med	high	
TOTAL CALORIES BURNED						

COMMENTS:

Type:
Qty:
Type:
Qty:
Type:
Qty:
Type:
Qty:
Type:
Qty:
Type:
Qty:

Daily Assessment and Notes

OBSTACLES, SOLUTIONS AND THOUGHTS ON YOUR PROGRESS

Daily Nutritional Intake

FOOD AND BEVERAGES

Don't be too hard
on yourself if you
happen to stumble
in your plan along
the way. Be sure
not to use it as an
excuse to stop
exercising or your
weight-loss
program.

Just remind your-
self that tomorrow
is another day, and
you can get back
on track.

MORNING TIME:	amt.	cal.	fat gms	protein gms	carbs. gms	fiber gms
BREAKFAST TOTALS						

COMMENTS:

AFTERNOON TIME:	amt.	cal.	fat gms	protein gms	carbs. gms	fiber gms
LUNCH TOTALS						

COMMENTS:

Daily Serving Intake

____ Fruits
# of servings

____ Vegetables
# of servings

____ Grains
# of servings

____ Meat & Beans
# of servings

____ Milk & Dairy
# of servings

____ Oils & Sweets
# of servings

EVENING TIME:	amt.	cal.	fat gms	protein gms	carbs. gms	fiber gms
DINNER TOTALS						

Water Intake

oz.

COMMENTS:

❏ low ❏ med ❏ high

ENERGY LEVELS

Daily Nutritional Intake

FOOD AND BEVERAGES

DAILY GOALS
ACHIEVED

SNACKS TIME:	amt.	cal.	fat gms	protein gms	carbs. gms	fiber gms
SNACK TOTALS						

COMMENTS:

DAILY TOTALS

Calories

Fat

Protein

Carbohydrates

Fiber

Other

Exercise and Fitness

DAILY PHYSICAL ACTIVITIES

ACTIVITY/ EXERCISE	hrs./ mins.	reps./ sets	------INTENSITY------			cal. burned
			low	med	high	
TOTAL CALORIES BURNED						

COMMENTS:

VITAMINS &
SUPPLEMENTS

Type:

Qty:

Type:

Qty:

Type:

Qty:

Type:

Qty:

Type:

Qty:

Type:

Qty:

Daily Assessment and Notes

OBSTACLES, SOLUTIONS AND THOUGHTS ON YOUR PROGRESS

DATE _____   **WEIGHT** _____

Daily Nutritional Intake

FOOD AND BEVERAGES

MORNING TIME:	amt.	cal.	fat gms	protein gms	carbs. gms	fiber gms
BREAKFAST TOTALS						

COMMENTS:

AFTERNOON TIME:	amt.	cal.	fat gms	protein gms	carbs. gms	fiber gms
LUNCH TOTALS						

COMMENTS:

EVENING TIME:	amt.	cal.	fat gms	protein gms	carbs. gms	fiber gms
DINNER TOTALS						

COMMENTS:

Helpful Tips for Effective Weight-Loss

If you have a lot of weight to lose, set temporary or short-term goals for yourself. Breaking the journey down into smaller sections can make it easier to stay on track.

Daily Serving Intake

_____ Fruits
# of servings

_____ Vegetables
# of servings

_____ Grains
# of servings

_____ Meat & Beans
# of servings

_____ Milk & Dairy
# of servings

_____ Oils & Sweets
# of servings

Water Intake

oz. _____

66

DAILY GOALS
ACHIEVED

Daily Nutritional Intake

FOOD AND BEVERAGES

DAILY TOTALS

SNACKS TIME:	amt.	cal.	fat gms	protein gms	carbs. gms	fiber gms
SNACK TOTALS						

COMMENTS:

Calories

Fat

Protein

Carbohydrates

Fiber

Other

Exercise and Fitness

DAILY PHYSICAL ACTIVITIES

VITAMINS &
SUPPLEMENTS

ACTIVITY/ EXERCISE	hrs./ mins.	reps./ sets	------INTENSITY------			cal. burned
			low	med	high	
TOTAL CALORIES BURNED						

COMMENTS:

Type:
Qty:
Type:
Qty:
Type:
Qty:
Type:
Qty:
Type:
Qty:
Type:
Qty:

Daily Assessment and Notes

OBSTACLES, SOLUTIONS AND THOUGHTS ON YOUR PROGRESS

Helpful Tips for Effective Weight-Loss

Finding a friend to share in your weight-loss journey can help you to remain on track and stay motivated. Having someone along to encourage and support you in your progress is a good way to maintain confidence in your plan.

Daily Nutritional Intake

FOOD AND BEVERAGES

MORNING TIME:	amt.	cal.	fat gms	protein gms	carbs. gms	fiber gms
BREAKFAST TOTALS						

COMMENTS:

AFTERNOON TIME:	amt.	cal.	fat gms	protein gms	carbs. gms	fiber gms
LUNCH TOTALS						

COMMENTS:

Daily Serving Intake

____ Fruits
# of servings

____ Vegetables
# of servings

____ Grains
# of servings

____ Meat & Beans
# of servings

____ Milk & Dairy
# of servings

____ Oils & Sweets
# of servings

Water Intake

oz.

EVENING TIME:	amt.	cal.	fat gms	protein gms	carbs. gms	fiber gms
DINNER TOTALS						

COMMENTS:

❑ low ❑ med ❑ high

ENERGY LEVELS

Daily Nutritional Intake

FOOD AND BEVERAGES

DAILY GOALS
ACHIEVED

DAILY TOTALS

SNACKS TIME:	amt.	cal.	fat gms	protein gms	carbs. gms	fiber gms
SNACK TOTALS						

COMMENTS:

Calories

Fat

Protein

Carbohydrates

Fiber

Other

Exercise and Fitness

DAILY PHYSICAL ACTIVITIES

VITAMINS &
SUPPLEMENTS

ACTIVITY/ EXERCISE	hrs./ mins.	reps./ sets	------INTENSITY------ low	med	high	cal. burned
TOTAL CALORIES BURNED						

COMMENTS:

Type:

Qty:

Type:

Qty:

Type:

Qty:

Type:

Qty:

Type:

Qty:

Type:

Qty:

Daily Assessment and Notes

OBSTACLES, SOLUTIONS AND THOUGHTS ON YOUR PROGRESS

WEIGHT

Helpful Tips
for Effective
Weight-Loss

Moderation is the
key to a healthy
lifestyle and to
losing weight.
Keep the portions
small on your plate,
using your hand as
a good guide for
how big or small
your portions of
food should be.

Daily Nutritional Intake

FOOD AND BEVERAGES

MORNING TIME:	amt.	cal.	fat gms	protein gms	carbs. gms	fiber gms
BREAKFAST TOTALS						

COMMENTS:

AFTERNOON TIME:	amt.	cal.	fat gms	protein gms	carbs. gms	fiber gms
LUNCH TOTALS						

COMMENTS:

Daily Serving Intake

_____ Fruits
# of servings

_____ Vegetables
# of servings

_____ Grains
# of servings

_____ Meat & Beans
# of servings

_____ Milk & Dairy
# of servings

_____ Oils & Sweets
# of servings

EVENING TIME:	amt.	cal.	fat gms	protein gms	carbs. gms	fiber gms
DINNER TOTALS						

Water Intake

oz. _____

COMMENTS:

☐ low ☐ med ☐ high

ENERGY LEVELS

Daily Nutritional Intake

FOOD AND BEVERAGES

DAILY GOALS
ACHIEVED

SNACKS TIME:	amt.	cal.	fat gms	protein gms	carbs. gms	fiber gms
SNACK TOTALS						

COMMENTS:

DAILY TOTALS

Calories

Fat

Protein

Carbohydrates

Fiber

Other

Exercise and Fitness

DAILY PHYSICAL ACTIVITIES

ACTIVITY/ EXERCISE	hrs./ mins.	reps./ sets	------INTENSITY------			cal. burned
			low	med	high	
TOTAL CALORIES BURNED						

COMMENTS:

VITAMINS &
SUPPLEMENTS

Type:
Qty:
Type:
Qty:
Type:
Qty:
Type:
Qty:
Type:
Qty:
Type:
Qty:

Daily Assessment and Notes

OBSTACLES, SOLUTIONS AND THOUGHTS ON YOUR PROGRESS

Helpful Tips
for Effective
Weight-Loss

Daily Nutritional Intake

FOOD AND BEVERAGES

Drink plenty of
water each day.
Often we think we
are hungry when
our body is sending
us signals that we
are actually thirsty
or dehydrated.
Keeping yourself
hydrated through-
out the day will
help prevent you
from eating when
you are not hungry.

MORNING TIME:	amt.	cal.	fat gms	protein gms	carbs. gms	fiber gms
BREAKFAST TOTALS						

COMMENTS:

AFTERNOON TIME:	amt.	cal.	fat gms	protein gms	carbs. gms	fiber gms
LUNCH TOTALS						

COMMENTS:

Daily Serving Intake

_____ Fruits
# of servings

_____ Vegetables
# of servings

_____ Grains
# of servings

_____ Meat & Beans
# of servings

_____ Milk & Dairy
# of servings

_____ Oils & Sweets
# of servings

Water Intake

oz.

EVENING TIME:	amt.	cal.	fat gms	protein gms	carbs. gms	fiber gms
DINNER TOTALS						

COMMENTS:

❏ low ❏ med ❏ high

ENERGY LEVELS

Daily Nutritional Intake

FOOD AND BEVERAGES

DAILY GOALS
ACHIEVED

SNACKS TIME:	amt.	cal.	fat gms	protein gms	carbs. gms	fiber gms
SNACK TOTALS						

COMMENTS:

DAILY TOTALS

Calories

Fat

Protein

Carbohydrates

Fiber

Other

Exercise and Fitness

DAILY PHYSICAL ACTIVITIES

ACTIVITY/ EXERCISE	hrs./ mins.	reps./ sets	------INTENSITY------ low	med	high	cal. burned
TOTAL CALORIES BURNED						

COMMENTS:

VITAMINS &
SUPPLEMENTS

Type:

Qty:

Type:

Qty:

Type:

Qty:

Type:

Qty:

Type:

Qty:

Type:

Qty:

Daily Assessment and Notes

OBSTACLES, SOLUTIONS AND THOUGHTS ON YOUR PROGRESS

Helpful Tips
for Effective
Weight-Loss

Cook meals at home as much as possible. Restaurant meals can contain hidden calories and fats, and often the portion sizes are too big for our own good. Meals made at home are healthier, and you can control how much you make and eat.

Daily Nutritional Intake

FOOD AND BEVERAGES

MORNING TIME:	amt.	cal.	fat gms	protein gms	carbs. gms	fiber gms
BREAKFAST TOTALS						

COMMENTS:

AFTERNOON TIME:	amt.	cal.	fat gms	protein gms	carbs. gms	fiber gms
LUNCH TOTALS						

COMMENTS:

Daily Serving Intake

_____ Fruits
# of servings

_____ Vegetables
# of servings

_____ Grains
# of servings

_____ Meat & Beans
# of servings

_____ Milk & Dairy
# of servings

_____ Oils & Sweets
# of servings

EVENING TIME:	amt.	cal.	fat gms	protein gms	carbs. gms	fiber gms
DINNER TOTALS						

Water Intake

oz.

COMMENTS:

☐ low ☐ med ☐ high

ENERGY LEVELS

Daily Nutritional Intake

FOOD AND BEVERAGES

DAILY GOALS ACHIEVED

SNACKS TIME:	amt.	cal.	fat gms	protein gms	carbs. gms	fiber gms
SNACK TOTALS						

COMMENTS:

DAILY TOTALS

Calories

Fat

Protein

Carbohydrates

Fiber

Other

Exercise and Fitness

DAILY PHYSICAL ACTIVITIES

ACTIVITY/ EXERCISE	hrs./ mins.	reps./ sets	------INTENSITY------			cal. burned
			low	med	high	
TOTAL CALORIES BURNED						

COMMENTS:

VITAMINS & SUPPLEMENTS

Type:

Qty:

Type:

Qty:

Type:

Qty:

Type:

Qty:

Type:

Qty:

Type:

Qty:

Daily Assessment and Notes

OBSTACLES, SOLUTIONS AND THOUGHTS ON YOUR PROGRESS

Helpful Tips
for Effective
Weight-Loss

Daily Nutritional Intake

FOOD AND BEVERAGES

Try to incorporate
a rainbow of colors
into your diet by
eating plenty of
vegetables and
fruits.

MORNING TIME:	amt.	cal.	fat gms	protein gms	carbs. gms	fiber gms
BREAKFAST TOTALS						

COMMENTS:

AFTERNOON TIME:	amt.	cal.	fat gms	protein gms	carbs. gms	fiber gms
LUNCH TOTALS						

COMMENTS:

Daily Serving Intake

____ Fruits
# of servings

____ Vegetables
# of servings

____ Grains
# of servings

____ Meat & Beans
# of servings

____ Milk & Dairy
# of servings

____ Oils & Sweets
# of servings

Water Intake

oz. ____

EVENING TIME:	amt.	cal.	fat gms	protein gms	carbs. gms	fiber gms
DINNER TOTALS						

COMMENTS:

☐ low ☐ med ☐ high

ENERGY LEVELS

Daily Nutritional Intake

FOOD AND BEVERAGES

**DAILY GOALS
ACHIEVED**

DAILY TOTALS

SNACKS		amt.	cal.	fat gms	protein gms	carbs. gms	fiber gms
TIME:							
SNACK TOTALS							

Calories

Fat

Protein

Carbohydrates

Fiber

Other

COMMENTS:

Exercise and Fitness

DAILY PHYSICAL ACTIVITIES

VITAMINS &

SUPPLEMENTS

ACTIVITY/	hrs./ mins.	reps./ sets	------INTENSITY------			cal. burned
EXERCISE			low	med	high	
TOTAL CALORIES BURNED						

Type:

Qty:

Type:

Qty:

Type:

Qty:

Type:

Qty:

Type:

Qty:

Type:

Qty:

COMMENTS:

Daily Assessment and Notes

OBSTACLES, SOLUTIONS AND THOUGHTS ON YOUR PROGRESS

Daily Nutritional Intake

FOOD AND BEVERAGES

Consult your
primary care
physician about the
types of supple-
ments you should
be taking while on
your diet. He or
she will be able to
tell you exactly
what vitamins and
minerals you
should be getting.

MORNING TIME:	amt.	cal.	fat gms	protein gms	carbs. gms	fiber gms
BREAKFAST TOTALS						

COMMENTS:

AFTERNOON TIME:	amt.	cal.	fat gms	protein gms	carbs. gms	fiber gms
LUNCH TOTALS						

COMMENTS:

Daily Serving Intake

_____ Fruits
# of servings

_____ Vegetables
# of servings

_____ Grains
# of servings

_____ Meat & Beans
# of servings

_____ Milk & Dairy
# of servings

_____ Oils & Sweets
# of servings

EVENING TIME:	amt.	cal.	fat gms	protein gms	carbs. gms	fiber gms
DINNER TOTALS						

Water Intake

oz.

COMMENTS:

❏ low   ❏ med   ❏ high

ENERGY LEVELS

Daily Nutritional Intake

FOOD AND BEVERAGES

**DAILY GOALS
ACHIEVED**

SNACKS TIME:	amt.	cal.	fat gms	protein gms	carbs. gms	fiber gms
SNACK TOTALS						

COMMENTS:

DAILY TOTALS

Calories

Fat

Protein

Carbohydrates

Fiber

Other

Exercise and Fitness

DAILY PHYSICAL ACTIVITIES

ACTIVITY/ EXERCISE	hrs./ mins.	reps./ sets	------INTENSITY------ low	med	high	cal. burned
TOTAL CALORIES BURNED						

COMMENTS:

**VITAMINS &
SUPPLEMENTS**

Type:

Qty:

Type:

Qty:

Type:

Qty:

Type:

Qty:

Type:

Qty:

Type:

Qty:

Daily Assessment and Notes

OBSTACLES, SOLUTIONS AND THOUGHTS ON YOUR PROGRESS

Helpful Tips
for Effective
Weight-Loss

Daily Nutritional Intake

FOOD AND BEVERAGES

Be realistic with
yourself. Make
your weight-loss
goals reasonable
and reachable; that
way you will be
more likely to reach
them and achieve
your resolutions.

MORNING TIME:	amt.	cal.	fat gms	protein gms	carbs. gms	fiber gms
BREAKFAST TOTALS						

COMMENTS:

AFTERNOON TIME:	amt.	cal.	fat gms	protein gms	carbs. gms	fiber gms
LUNCH TOTALS						

COMMENTS:

Daily Serving Intake

____ Fruits
# of servings

____ Vegetables
# of servings

____ Grains
# of servings

____ Meat & Beans
# of servings

____ Milk & Dairy
# of servings

____ Oils & Sweets
# of servings

Water Intake

oz.

EVENING TIME:	amt.	cal.	fat gms	protein gms	carbs. gms	fiber gms
DINNER TOTALS						

COMMENTS:

❑ low   ❑ med   ❑ high

ENERGY LEVELS

Daily Nutritional Intake

FOOD AND BEVERAGES

DAILY GOALS
ACHIEVED

SNACKS TIME:	amt.	cal.	fat gms	protein gms	carbs. gms	fiber gms
SNACK TOTALS						

COMMENTS:

DAILY TOTALS

Calories

Fat

Protein

Carbohydrates

Fiber

Other

Exercise and Fitness

DAILY PHYSICAL ACTIVITIES

ACTIVITY/ EXERCISE	hrs./ mins.	reps./ sets	------INTENSITY------			cal. burned
			low	med	high	
TOTAL CALORIES BURNED						

COMMENTS:

VITAMINS &
SUPPLEMENTS

Type:
Qty:
Type:
Qty:
Type:
Qty:
Type:
Qty:
Type:
Qty:
Type:
Qty:

Daily Assessment and Notes

OBSTACLES, SOLUTIONS AND THOUGHTS ON YOUR PROGRESS

Daily Nutritional Intake

FOOD AND BEVERAGES

MORNING TIME:	amt.	cal.	fat gms	protein gms	carbs. gms	fiber gms
BREAKFAST TOTALS						

COMMENTS:

AFTERNOON TIME:	amt.	cal.	fat gms	protein gms	carbs. gms	fiber gms
LUNCH TOTALS						

COMMENTS:

EVENING TIME:	amt.	cal.	fat gms	protein gms	carbs. gms	fiber gms
DINNER TOTALS						

COMMENTS:

Daily Serving Intake

_____ Fruits
# of servings

_____ Vegetables
# of servings

_____ Grains
# of servings

_____ Meat & Beans
# of servings

_____ Milk & Dairy
# of servings

_____ Oils & Sweets
# of servings

Water Intake

oz.

☐ low ☐ med ☐ high

ENERGY LEVELS

Daily Nutritional Intake

FOOD AND BEVERAGES

DAILY GOALS
ACHIEVED

SNACKS TIME:	amt.	cal.	fat gms	protein gms	carbs. gms	fiber gms
SNACK TOTALS						

COMMENTS:

DAILY TOTALS

Calories

Fat

Protein

Carbohydrates

Fiber

Other

Exercise and Fitness

DAILY PHYSICAL ACTIVITIES

ACTIVITY/ EXERCISE	hrs./ mins.	reps./ sets	------INTENSITY------ low	med	high	cal. burned
TOTAL CALORIES BURNED						

COMMENTS:

VITAMINS &
SUPPLEMENTS

Type:

Qty:

Type:

Qty:

Type:

Qty:

Type:

Qty:

Type:

Qty:

Type:

Qty:

Daily Assessment and Notes

OBSTACLES, SOLUTIONS AND THOUGHTS ON YOUR PROGRESS

Daily Nutritional Intake

FOOD AND BEVERAGES

MORNING TIME:	amt.	cal.	fat gms	protein gms	carbs. gms	fiber gms
BREAKFAST TOTALS						

COMMENTS:

AFTERNOON TIME:	amt.	cal.	fat gms	protein gms	carbs. gms	fiber gms
LUNCH TOTALS						

COMMENTS:

Daily Serving Intake

____ Fruits
   # of servings

____ Vegetables
   # of servings

____ Grains
   # of servings

____ Meat & Beans
   # of servings

____ Milk & Dairy
   # of servings

____ Oils & Sweets
   # of servings

EVENING TIME:	amt.	cal.	fat gms	protein gms	carbs. gms	fiber gms
DINNER TOTALS						

COMMENTS:

Water Intake

oz.

**DAILY GOALS
ACHIEVED**

Daily Nutritional Intake

FOOD AND BEVERAGES

SNACKS TIME:	amt.	cal.	fat gms	protein gms	carbs. gms	fiber gms
SNACK TOTALS						

COMMENTS:

DAILY TOTALS

Calories

Fat

Protein

Carbohydrates

Fiber

Other

Exercise and Fitness

DAILY PHYSICAL ACTIVITIES

ACTIVITY/ EXERCISE	hrs./ mins.	reps./ sets	------INTENSITY------			cal. burned
			low	med	high	
TOTAL CALORIES BURNED						

COMMENTS:

**VITAMINS &
SUPPLEMENTS**

Type:

Qty:

Type:

Qty:

Type:

Qty:

Type:

Qty:

Type:

Qty:

Type:

Qty:

Daily Assessment and Notes

OBSTACLES, SOLUTIONS AND THOUGHTS ON YOUR PROGRESS

WEIGHT

Helpful Tips
for Effective
Weight-Loss

Daily Nutritional Intake

FOOD AND BEVERAGES

Whole grains can
be very beneficial
to your body. They
can help reduce the
risk of high choles-
terol or blood pres-
sure, diabetes, and
certain heart dis-
eases.

Try to incorporate
a good amount of
whole grains into
your diet to keep
your body strong
against these types
of diseases.

MORNING TIME:	amt.	cal.	fat gms	protein gms	carbs. gms	fiber gms
BREAKFAST TOTALS						

COMMENTS:

AFTERNOON TIME:	amt.	cal.	fat gms	protein gms	carbs. gms	fiber gms
LUNCH TOTALS						

COMMENTS:

Daily Serving Intake

_____ Fruits
      # of servings

_____ Vegetables
      # of servings

_____ Grains
      # of servings

_____ Meat & Beans
      # of servings

_____ Milk & Dairy
      # of servings

_____ Oils & Sweets
      # of servings

Water Intake

oz.

EVENING TIME:	amt.	cal.	fat gms	protein gms	carbs. gms	fiber gms
DINNER TOTALS						

COMMENTS:

❑ low ❑ med ❑ high

ENERGY LEVELS

Daily Nutritional Intake

FOOD AND BEVERAGES

DAILY GOALS
ACHIEVED

SNACKS TIME:	amt.	cal.	fat gms	protein gms	carbs. gms	fiber gms
SNACK TOTALS						

COMMENTS:

DAILY TOTALS

Calories

Fat

Protein

Carbohydrates

Fiber

Other

Exercise and Fitness

DAILY PHYSICAL ACTIVITIES

ACTIVITY/ EXERCISE	hrs./ mins.	reps./ sets	------INTENSITY------			cal. burned
			low	med	high	
TOTAL CALORIES BURNED						

COMMENTS:

VITAMINS &

SUPPLEMENTS

Type:

Qty:

Type:

Qty:

Type:

Qty:

Type:

Qty:

Type:

Qty:

Type:

Qty:

Daily Assessment and Notes

OBSTACLES, SOLUTIONS AND THOUGHTS ON YOUR PROGRESS

WEIGHT

**Helpful Tips
for Effective
Weight-Loss**

Achieving a healthy
lifestyle takes time
and practice, but
you can do it.

Establish good
eating habits so you
can make healthy
choices for your
diet. Keep physical
fitness a priority
through exercise
routines that are
realistic, maintain-
able, and fun.

Daily Serving Intake

____ Fruits
# of servings

____ Vegetables
# of servings

____ Grains
# of servings

____ Meat & Beans
# of servings

____ Milk & Dairy
# of servings

____ Oils & Sweets
# of servings

Water Intake

oz. _____

88

Daily Nutritional Intake

FOOD AND BEVERAGES

MORNING TIME:	amt.	cal.	fat gms	protein gms	carbs. gms	fiber gms
BREAKFAST TOTALS						

COMMENTS:

AFTERNOON TIME:	amt.	cal.	fat gms	protein gms	carbs. gms	fiber gms
LUNCH TOTALS						

COMMENTS:

EVENING TIME:	amt.	cal.	fat gms	protein gms	carbs. gms	fiber gms
DINNER TOTALS						

COMMENTS:

❑ low ❑ med ❑ high

ENERGY LEVELS

Daily Nutritional Intake

FOOD AND BEVERAGES

**DAILY GOALS
ACHIEVED**

DAILY TOTALS

SNACKS TIME:	amt.	cal.	fat gms	protein gms	carbs. gms	fiber gms
SNACK TOTALS						

COMMENTS:

Calories

Fat

Protein

Carbohydrates

Fiber

Other

Exercise and Fitness

DAILY PHYSICAL ACTIVITIES

**VITAMINS &
SUPPLEMENTS**

ACTIVITY/ EXERCISE	hrs./ mins.	reps./ sets	------INTENSITY------			cal. burned
			low	med	high	
TOTAL CALORIES BURNED						

COMMENTS:

Type:
Qty:
Type:
Qty:
Type:
Qty:
Type:
Qty:
Type:
Qty:
Type:
Qty:

Daily Assessment and Notes

OBSTACLES, SOLUTIONS AND THOUGHTS ON YOUR PROGRESS

**Helpful Tips
for Effective
Weight-Loss**

If you cannot make
it to the gym every
day, try to incorpo-
rate other physical
activities into your
day, such as gar-
dening, vacuuming
or shopping.

Combining a few of
these activities can
be the equivalent of
spending a couple
of hours in the
gym.

Daily Serving Intake

_____ Fruits
       # of servings

_____ Vegetables
       # of servings

_____ Grains
       # of servings

_____ Meat & Beans
       # of servings

_____ Milk & Dairy
       # of servings

_____ Oils & Sweets
       # of servings

Water Intake

_____ # oz.

Daily Nutritional Intake

FOOD AND BEVERAGES

MORNING TIME:	amt.	cal.	fat gms	protein gms	carbs. gms	fiber gms
BREAKFAST TOTALS						

COMMENTS:

AFTERNOON TIME:	amt.	cal.	fat gms	protein gms	carbs. gms	fiber gms
LUNCH TOTALS						

COMMENTS:

EVENING TIME:	amt.	cal.	fat gms	protein gms	carbs. gms	fiber gms
DINNER TOTALS						

COMMENTS:

Daily Nutritional Intake

FOOD AND BEVERAGES

DAILY GOALS
ACHIEVED

DAILY TOTALS

SNACKS TIME:	amt.	cal.	fat gms	protein gms	carbs. gms	fiber gms
SNACK TOTALS						

COMMENTS:

Calories

Fat

Protein

Carbohydrates

Fiber

Other

Exercise and Fitness

DAILY PHYSICAL ACTIVITIES

VITAMINS &
SUPPLEMENTS

ACTIVITY/ EXERCISE	hrs./ mins.	reps./ sets	low	med	high	cal. burned
TOTAL CALORIES BURNED						

INTENSITY (spanning low, med, high)

COMMENTS:

Type:
Qty:
Type:
Qty:
Type:
Qty:
Type:
Qty:
Type:
Qty:
Type:
Qty:

Daily Assessment and Notes

OBSTACLES, SOLUTIONS AND THOUGHTS ON YOUR PROGRESS

Helpful Tips
for Effective
Weight-Loss

Exercise helps you
lose weight by rais-
ing your metabo-
lism so you contin-
ue burning excess
calories for several
hours after you fin-
ish exercising.
Only activities that
increase your body
temperature and
make you sweat
will increase your
metabolism enough
to continue burning
more calories after
you finish.

Daily Nutritional Intake

FOOD AND BEVERAGES

MORNING TIME:	amt.	cal.	fat gms	protein gms	carbs. gms	fiber gms
BREAKFAST TOTALS						

COMMENTS:

AFTERNOON TIME:	amt.	cal.	fat gms	protein gms	carbs. gms	fiber gms
LUNCH TOTALS						

COMMENTS:

EVENING TIME:	amt.	cal.	fat gms	protein gms	carbs. gms	fiber gms
DINNER TOTALS						

COMMENTS:

Daily Serving Intake

_____ Fruits
# of servings

_____ Vegetables
# of servings

_____ Grains
# of servings

_____ Meat & Beans
# of servings

_____ Milk & Dairy
# of servings

_____ Oils & Sweets
# of servings

Water Intake

oz.

☐ low   ☐ med   ☐ high

ENERGY LEVELS

Daily Nutritional Intake

FOOD AND BEVERAGES

DAILY GOALS
ACHIEVED

SNACKS TIME:	amt.	cal.	fat gms	protein gms	carbs. gms	fiber gms
SNACK TOTALS						

COMMENTS:

DAILY TOTALS

Calories

Fat

Protein

Carbohydrates

Fiber

Other

Exercise and Fitness

DAILY PHYSICAL ACTIVITIES

VITAMINS &
SUPPLEMENTS

ACTIVITY/ EXERCISE	hrs./ mins.	reps./ sets	------INTENSITY------ low	med	high	cal. burned
TOTAL CALORIES BURNED						

COMMENTS:

Type:

Qty:

Type:

Qty:

Type:

Qty:

Type:

Qty:

Type:

Qty:

Type:

Qty:

Daily Assessment and Notes

OBSTACLES, SOLUTIONS AND THOUGHTS ON YOUR PROGRESS

Helpful Tips
for Effective
Weight-Loss

When dining out,
be aware of hidden
calories, sodium,
and fats that could
be included in
sauces or the way
the meals are pre-
pared in the
kitchen.

Don't be afraid to
ask your server
how the meal is
prepared, or to
request the food be
prepared in a way
that is in order
with your diet pro-
gram.

Daily Serving Intake

____ Fruits
 # of servings

____ Vegetables
 # of servings

____ Grains
 # of servings

____ Meat & Beans
 # of servings

____ Milk & Dairy
 # of servings

____ Oils & Sweets
 # of servings

Water Intake

oz.

Daily Nutritional Intake

FOOD AND BEVERAGES

MORNING TIME:		amt.	cal.	fat gms	protein gms	carbs. gms	fiber gms
BREAKFAST TOTALS							

COMMENTS:

AFTERNOON TIME:		amt.	cal.	fat gms	protein gms	carbs. gms	fiber gms
LUNCH TOTALS							

COMMENTS:

EVENING TIME:		amt.	cal.	fat gms	protein gms	carbs. gms	fiber gms
DINNER TOTALS							

COMMENTS:

ENERGY LEVELS

Daily Nutritional Intake

FOOD AND BEVERAGES

**DAILY GOALS
ACHIEVED**

SNACKS TIME:	amt.	cal.	fat gms	protein gms	carbs. gms	fiber gms
SNACK TOTALS						

COMMENTS:

DAILY TOTALS

Calories

Fat

Protein

Carbohydrates

Fiber

Other

Exercise and Fitness

DAILY PHYSICAL ACTIVITIES

ACTIVITY/ EXERCISE	hrs./ mins.	reps./ sets	------INTENSITY------ low	med	high	cal. burned
TOTAL CALORIES BURNED						

COMMENTS:

VITAMINS &

SUPPLEMENTS

Type:

Qty:

Type:

Qty:

Type:

Qty:

Type:

Qty:

Type:

Qty:

Type:

Qty:

Daily Assessment and Notes

OBSTACLES, SOLUTIONS AND THOUGHTS ON YOUR PROGRESS

DATE   **WEIGHT**

Daily Nutritional Intake

FOOD AND BEVERAGES

**Helpful Tips
for Effective
Weight-Loss**

Restaurant portions
these days can
often be more food
than you need. Try
to eat only part of
what is on your
plate, and get a box
or bag to take the
rest home with you.

MORNING TIME:	amt.	cal.	fat gms	protein gms	carbs. gms	fiber gms
BREAKFAST TOTALS						

COMMENTS:

AFTERNOON TIME:	amt.	cal.	fat gms	protein gms	carbs. gms	fiber gms
LUNCH TOTALS						

COMMENTS:

Daily Serving Intake

_____ Fruits
     # of servings

_____ Vegetables
     # of servings

_____ Grains
     # of servings

_____ Meat & Beans
     # of servings

_____ Milk & Dairy
     # of servings

_____ Oils & Sweets
     # of servings

Water Intake

oz.

EVENING TIME:	amt.	cal.	fat gms	protein gms	carbs. gms	fiber gms
DINNER TOTALS						

COMMENTS:

❏ low ❏ med ❏ high

ENERGY LEVELS

Daily Nutritional Intake

FOOD AND BEVERAGES

DAILY GOALS
ACHIEVED

SNACKS TIME:	amt.	cal.	fat gms	protein gms	carbs. gms	fiber gms
SNACK TOTALS						

COMMENTS:

DAILY TOTALS

Calories

Fat

Protein

Carbohydrates

Fiber

Other

Exercise and Fitness

DAILY PHYSICAL ACTIVITIES

ACTIVITY/ EXERCISE	hrs./ mins.	reps./ sets	------INTENSITY------ low	med	high	cal. burned
TOTAL CALORIES BURNED						

COMMENTS:

VITAMINS &
SUPPLEMENTS

Type:

Qty:

Type:

Qty:

Type:

Qty:

Type:

Qty:

Type:

Qty:

Type:

Qty:

Daily Assessment and Notes

OBSTACLES, SOLUTIONS AND THOUGHTS ON YOUR PROGRESS

Daily Nutritional Intake

FOOD AND BEVERAGES

MORNING TIME:	amt.	cal.	fat gms	protein gms	carbs. gms	fiber gms
BREAKFAST TOTALS						

COMMENTS:

AFTERNOON TIME:	amt.	cal.	fat gms	protein gms	carbs. gms	fiber gms
LUNCH TOTALS						

COMMENTS:

EVENING TIME:	amt.	cal.	fat gms	protein gms	carbs. gms	fiber gms
DINNER TOTALS						

COMMENTS:

Daily Serving Intake

____ Fruits
# of servings

____ Vegetables
# of servings

____ Grains
# of servings

____ Meat & Beans
# of servings

____ Milk & Dairy
# of servings

____ Oils & Sweets
# of servings

Water Intake

oz.

☐ low ☐ med ☐ high

ENERGY LEVELS

Daily Nutritional Intake

FOOD AND BEVERAGES

SNACKS TIME:	amt.	cal.	fat gms	protein gms	carbs. gms	fiber gms
SNACK TOTALS						

COMMENTS:

DAILY TOTALS

Calories

Fat

Protein

Carbohydrates

Fiber

Other

Exercise and Fitness

DAILY PHYSICAL ACTIVITIES

ACTIVITY/ EXERCISE	hrs./ mins.	reps./ sets	------INTENSITY------			cal. burned
			low	med	high	
TOTAL CALORIES BURNED						

COMMENTS:

VITAMINS &
SUPPLEMENTS

Type:
Qty:
Type:
Qty:
Type:
Qty:
Type:
Qty:
Type:
Qty:
Type:
Qty:
Type:
Qty:

Daily Assessment and Notes

OBSTACLES, SOLUTIONS AND THOUGHTS ON YOUR PROGRESS

WEIGHT

Helpful Tips
for Effective
Weight-Loss

When you want
sound nutrition
information, con-
sider consulting a
registered dietitian,
or RD.

He or she will be a
highly trained food
and nutrition
expert who can
help you with your
nutrition questions.

Daily Nutritional Intake

FOOD AND BEVERAGES

MORNING TIME:	amt.	cal.	fat gms	protein gms	carbs. gms	fiber gms
BREAKFAST TOTALS						

COMMENTS:

AFTERNOON TIME:	amt.	cal.	fat gms	protein gms	carbs. gms	fiber gms
LUNCH TOTALS						

COMMENTS:

EVENING TIME:	amt.	cal.	fat gms	protein gms	carbs. gms	fiber gms
DINNER TOTALS						

COMMENTS:

Daily Serving Intake

____ Fruits
# of servings

____ Vegetables
# of servings

____ Grains
# of servings

____ Meat & Beans
# of servings

____ Milk & Dairy
# of servings

____ Oils & Sweets
# of servings

Water Intake

oz.

100

❏ low ❏ med ❏ high

ENERGY LEVELS

Daily Nutritional Intake

FOOD AND BEVERAGES

DAILY GOALS
ACHIEVED

SNACKS TIME:	amt.	cal.	fat gms	protein gms	carbs. gms	fiber gms
SNACK TOTALS						

COMMENTS:

DAILY TOTALS

Calories

Fat

Protein

Carbohydrates

Fiber

Other

Exercise and Fitness

DAILY PHYSICAL ACTIVITIES

ACTIVITY/ EXERCISE	hrs./ mins.	reps./ sets	------INTENSITY------ low	med	high	cal. burned
TOTAL CALORIES BURNED						

COMMENTS:

**VITAMINS &
SUPPLEMENTS**

Type:

Qty:

Type:

Qty:

Type:

Qty:

Type:

Qty:

Type:

Qty:

Type:

Qty:

Daily Assessment and Notes

OBSTACLES, SOLUTIONS AND THOUGHTS ON YOUR PROGRESS

DATE   **WEIGHT**

Helpful Tips
for Effective
Weight-Loss

Your weight-loss
plan can help you
create healthy
habits that last a
lifetime. Weight-
loss will help lower
your risk of certain
diseases, improve
your overall health,
and build your self-
confidence.

Daily Nutritional Intake

FOOD AND BEVERAGES

MORNING TIME:		amt.	cal.	fat gms	protein gms	carbs. gms	fiber gms
BREAKFAST TOTALS							

COMMENTS:

AFTERNOON TIME:		amt.	cal.	fat gms	protein gms	carbs. gms	fiber gms
LUNCH TOTALS							

COMMENTS:

Daily Serving Intake

_____ Fruits
# of servings

_____ Vegetables
# of servings

_____ Grains
# of servings

_____ Meat & Beans
# of servings

_____ Milk & Dairy
# of servings

_____ Oils & Sweets
# of servings

EVENING TIME:		amt.	cal.	fat gms	protein gms	carbs. gms	fiber gms
DINNER TOTALS							

COMMENTS:

Water Intake

oz.

102

❏ low ❏ med ❏ high

ENERGY LEVELS

Daily Nutritional Intake

FOOD AND BEVERAGES

DAILY GOALS
ACHIEVED

SNACKS TIME:	amt.	cal.	fat gms	protein gms	carbs. gms	fiber gms
SNACK TOTALS						

COMMENTS:

DAILY TOTALS

Calories

Fat

Protein

Carbohydrates

Fiber

Other

Exercise and Fitness

DAILY PHYSICAL ACTIVITIES

ACTIVITY/ EXERCISE	hrs./ mins.	reps./ sets	------INTENSITY------ low	med	high	cal. burned
TOTAL CALORIES BURNED						

COMMENTS:

VITAMINS &
SUPPLEMENTS

Type:

Qty:

Type:

Qty:

Type:

Qty:

Type:

Qty:

Type:

Qty:

Type:

Qty:

Daily Assessment and Notes

OBSTACLES, SOLUTIONS AND THOUGHTS ON YOUR PROGRESS

DATE

Daily Nutritional Intake

FOOD AND BEVERAGES

Helpful Tips
for Effective
Weight-Loss

If having a cookout
or barbeque,
choose lean cuts of
meat that have less
fat or trim off
excess fat before
cooking. They will
be a healthy choice
for you and your
guests, and taste
great!

MORNING TIME:	amt.	cal.	fat gms	protein gms	carbs. gms	fiber gms
BREAKFAST TOTALS						

COMMENTS:

AFTERNOON TIME:	amt.	cal.	fat gms	protein gms	carbs. gms	fiber gms
LUNCH TOTALS						

COMMENTS:

Daily Serving Intake

____ Fruits
# of servings

____ Vegetables
# of servings

____ Grains
# of servings

____ Meat & Beans
# of servings

____ Milk & Dairy
# of servings

____ Oils & Sweets
# of servings

Water Intake

___ oz.

EVENING TIME:	amt.	cal.	fat gms	protein gms	carbs. gms	fiber gms
DINNER TOTALS						

COMMENTS:

☐ low ☐ med ☐ high

ENERGY LEVELS

Daily Nutritional Intake

FOOD AND BEVERAGES

DAILY GOALS
ACHIEVED

SNACKS TIME:	amt.	cal.	fat gms	protein gms	carbs. gms	fiber gms
SNACK TOTALS						

COMMENTS:

DAILY TOTALS

Calories

Fat

Protein

Carbohydrates

Fiber

Other

Exercise and Fitness

DAILY PHYSICAL ACTIVITIES

ACTIVITY/ EXERCISE	hrs./ mins.	reps./ sets	low	med	high	cal. burned
TOTAL CALORIES BURNED						

COMMENTS:

VITAMINS &
SUPPLEMENTS

Type:

Qty:

Type:

Qty:

Type:

Qty:

Type:

Qty:

Type:

Qty:

Type:

Qty:

Daily Assessment and Notes

OBSTACLES, SOLUTIONS AND THOUGHTS ON YOUR PROGRESS

**Helpful Tips
for Effective
Weight-Loss**

Olive oil can add
flavor to any meal,
but be careful to
use it only in mod-
eration. No matter
what type of oil
you use, they are
all high in fat and
calories, so be sure
to go easy on the
portions.

Daily Nutritional Intake

FOOD AND BEVERAGES

MORNING TIME:	amt.	cal.	fat gms	protein gms	carbs. gms	fiber gms
BREAKFAST TOTALS						

COMMENTS:

AFTERNOON TIME:	amt.	cal.	fat gms	protein gms	carbs. gms	fiber gms
LUNCH TOTALS						

COMMENTS:

Daily Serving Intake

____ Fruits
# of servings

____ Vegetables
# of servings

____ Grains
# of servings

____ Meat & Beans
# of servings

____ Milk & Dairy
# of servings

____ Oils & Sweets
# of servings

Water Intake

oz.

EVENING TIME:	amt.	cal.	fat gms	protein gms	carbs. gms	fiber gms
DINNER TOTALS						

COMMENTS:

❑ low ❑ med ❑ high

ENERGY LEVELS

Daily Nutritional Intake

FOOD AND BEVERAGES

DAILY GOALS
ACHIEVED

SNACKS TIME:	amt.	cal.	fat gms	protein gms	carbs. gms	fiber gms
SNACK TOTALS						

COMMENTS:

DAILY TOTALS

Calories

Fat

Protein

Carbohydrates

Fiber

Other

Exercise and Fitness

DAILY PHYSICAL ACTIVITIES

VITAMINS &
SUPPLEMENTS

ACTIVITY/ EXERCISE	hrs./ mins.	reps./ sets	------INTENSITY------ low	med	high	cal. burned
TOTAL CALORIES BURNED						

COMMENTS:

Type:
Qty:
Type:
Qty:
Type:
Qty:
Type:
Qty:
Type:
Qty:
Type:
Qty:

Daily Assessment and Notes

OBSTACLES, SOLUTIONS AND THOUGHTS ON YOUR PROGRESS

107

Helpful Tips for Effective Weight-Loss

Caffeine can give you that boost you need to wake up in the morning, but it can trick your body into thinking it is hungry when it is not.

Make the switch from sodas and coffee to water by gradually reducing the amount of caffeine you consume each day.

Daily Serving Intake

____ Fruits
# of servings

____ Vegetables
# of servings

____ Grains
# of servings

____ Meat & Beans
# of servings

____ Milk & Dairy
# of servings

____ Oils & Sweets
# of servings

Water Intake

oz.

Daily Nutritional Intake

FOOD AND BEVERAGES

MORNING TIME:	amt.	cal.	fat gms	protein gms	carbs. gms	fiber gms
BREAKFAST TOTALS						

COMMENTS:

AFTERNOON TIME:	amt.	cal.	fat gms	protein gms	carbs. gms	fiber gms
LUNCH TOTALS						

COMMENTS:

EVENING TIME:	amt.	cal.	fat gms	protein gms	carbs. gms	fiber gms
DINNER TOTALS						

COMMENTS:

❏ low ❏ med ❏ high

ENERGY LEVELS

Daily Nutritional Intake

FOOD AND BEVERAGES

SNACKS TIME:	amt.	cal.	fat gms	protein gms	carbs. gms	fiber gms
SNACK TOTALS						
COMMENTS:						

DAILY TOTALS

Calories

Fat

Protein

Carbohydrates

Fiber

Other

Exercise and Fitness

DAILY PHYSICAL ACTIVITIES

VITAMINS &
SUPPLEMENTS

ACTIVITY/ EXERCISE	hrs./ mins.	reps./ sets	------INTENSITY------			cal. burned
			low	med	high	
TOTAL CALORIES BURNED						
COMMENTS:						

Type:
Qty:
Type:
Qty:
Type:
Qty:
Type:
Qty:
Type:
Qty:
Type:
Qty:

Daily Assessment and Notes

OBSTACLES, SOLUTIONS AND THOUGHTS ON YOUR PROGRESS

Daily Nutritional Intake

FOOD AND BEVERAGES

MORNING TIME:	amt.	cal.	fat gms	protein gms	carbs. gms	fiber gms
BREAKFAST TOTALS						

COMMENTS:

AFTERNOON TIME:	amt.	cal.	fat gms	protein gms	carbs. gms	fiber gms
LUNCH TOTALS						

COMMENTS:

Daily Serving Intake

_____ Fruits
# of servings

_____ Vegetables
# of servings

_____ Grains
# of servings

_____ Meat & Beans
# of servings

_____ Milk & Dairy
# of servings

_____ Oils & Sweets
# of servings

EVENING TIME:	amt.	cal.	fat gms	protein gms	carbs. gms	fiber gms
DINNER TOTALS						

COMMENTS:

Water Intake

oz.

❑ low ❑ med ❑ high
ENERGY LEVELS

Daily Nutritional Intake
FOOD AND BEVERAGES

DAILY GOALS
ACHIEVED

DAILY TOTALS

SNACKS TIME:	amt.	cal.	fat gms	protein gms	carbs. gms	fiber gms
SNACK TOTALS						

COMMENTS:

Calories

Fat

Protein

Carbohydrates

Fiber

Other

Exercise and Fitness
DAILY PHYSICAL ACTIVITIES

VITAMINS &
SUPPLEMENTS

ACTIVITY/ EXERCISE	hrs./ mins.	reps./ sets	------INTENSITY------			cal. burned
			low	med	high	
TOTAL CALORIES BURNED						

COMMENTS:

Type:

Qty:

Type:

Qty:

Type:

Qty:

Type:

Qty:

Type:

Qty:

Type:

Qty:

Daily Assessment and Notes
OBSTACLES, SOLUTIONS AND THOUGHTS ON YOUR PROGRESS

WEIGHT

Daily Nutritional Intake

FOOD AND BEVERAGES

If you are always
on-the-go, travel-
ing, or on vacation,
take time to pack
healthy snacks for
yourself to avoid
having limited
options. Consider
trail mix, dried
fruits, nuts, or
healthy crackers.

MORNING TIME:	amt.	cal.	fat gms	protein gms	carbs. gms	fiber gms
BREAKFAST TOTALS						

COMMENTS:

AFTERNOON TIME:	amt.	cal.	fat gms	protein gms	carbs. gms	fiber gms
LUNCH TOTALS						

COMMENTS:

Daily Serving Intake

_____ Fruits
         # of servings

_____ Vegetables
         # of servings

_____ Grains
         # of servings

_____ Meat & Beans
         # of servings

_____ Milk & Dairy
         # of servings

_____ Oils & Sweets
         # of servings

Water Intake

oz.

EVENING TIME:	amt.	cal.	fat gms	protein gms	carbs. gms	fiber gms
DINNER TOTALS						

COMMENTS:

☐ low ☐ med ☐ high

NERGY LEVELS

)aily Nutritional Intake

OOD AND BEVERAGES

SNACKS TIME:	amt.	cal.	fat gms	protein gms	carbs. gms	fiber gms
SNACK TOTALS						

COMMENTS:

DAILY TOTALS

Calories

Fat

Protein

Carbohydrates

Fiber

Other

Exercise and Fitness

DAILY PHYSICAL ACTIVITIES

ACTIVITY/ EXERCISE	hrs./ mins.	reps./ sets	low	med	high	cal. burned
TOTAL CALORIES BURNED						

------INTENSITY------

COMMENTS:

VITAMINS & SUPPLEMENTS

Type:

Qty:

Type:

Qty:

Type:

Qty:

Type:

Qty:

Type:

Qty:

Type:

Qty:

)aily Assessment and Notes

OBSTACLES, SOLUTIONS AND THOUGHTS ON YOUR PROGRESS

Daily Nutritional Intake

FOOD AND BEVERAGES

MORNING TIME:	amt.	cal.	fat gms	protein gms	carbs. gms	fiber gms
BREAKFAST TOTALS						

COMMENTS:

AFTERNOON TIME:	amt.	cal.	fat gms	protein gms	carbs. gms	fiber gms
LUNCH TOTALS						

COMMENTS:

Daily Serving Intake

____ Fruits
# of servings

____ Vegetables
# of servings

____ Grains
# of servings

____ Meat & Beans
# of servings

____ Milk & Dairy
# of servings

____ Oils & Sweets
# of servings

EVENING TIME:	amt.	cal.	fat gms	protein gms	carbs. gms	fiber gms
DINNER TOTALS						

COMMENTS:

Water Intake

oz.

ENERGY LEVELS

Daily Nutritional Intake

FOOD AND BEVERAGES

**DAILY GOALS
ACHIEVED**

SNACKS TIME:	amt.	cal.	fat gms	protein gms	carbs. gms	fiber gms
SNACK TOTALS						

COMMENTS:

DAILY TOTALS

Calories

Fat

Protein

Carbohydrates

Fiber

Other

Exercise and Fitness

DAILY PHYSICAL ACTIVITIES

ACTIVITY/ EXERCISE	hrs./ mins.	reps./ sets	low	med	high	cal. burned
TOTAL CALORIES BURNED						

------INTENSITY------ (low, med, high)

COMMENTS:

**VITAMINS &
SUPPLEMENTS**

Type:
Qty:
Type:
Qty:
Type:
Qty:
Type:
Qty:
Type:
Qty:
Type:
Qty:

Daily Assessment and Notes

OBSTACLES, SOLUTIONS AND THOUGHTS ON YOUR PROGRESS

WEIGHT

Daily Nutritional Intake

Helpful Tips for Effective Weight-Loss

Bottled fruit juice often contains a lot of sugars, so you end up consuming more calories than you need.

Try to stick with eating whole fruits, or else check the labels and make sure the juice you are drinking is 100% fruit juice. To reduce calories, you can also dilute fruit juice with water.

Daily Serving Intake

_____ Fruits
# of servings

_____ Vegetables
# of servings

_____ Grains
# of servings

_____ Meat & Beans
# of servings

_____ Milk & Dairy
# of servings

_____ Oils & Sweets
# of servings

Water Intake

oz.

FOOD AND BEVERAGES

MORNING TIME:	amt.	cal.	fat gms	protein gms	carbs. gms	fiber gms
BREAKFAST TOTALS						

COMMENTS:

AFTERNOON TIME:	amt.	cal.	fat gms	protein gms	carbs. gms	fiber gms
LUNCH TOTALS						

COMMENTS:

EVENING TIME:	amt.	cal.	fat gms	protein gms	carbs. gms	fiber gms
DINNER TOTALS						

COMMENTS:

❏ low ❏ med ❏ high

ENERGY LEVELS

Daily Nutritional Intake

FOOD AND BEVERAGES

DAILY GOALS ACHIEVED

DAILY TOTALS

SNACKS TIME:	amt.	cal.	fat gms	protein gms	carbs. gms	fiber gms
SNACK TOTALS						

COMMENTS:

Calories

Fat

Protein

Carbohydrates

Fiber

Other

Exercise and Fitness

DAILY PHYSICAL ACTIVITIES

VITAMINS & SUPPLEMENTS

ACTIVITY/ EXERCISE	hrs./ mins.	reps./ sets	------INTENSITY------			cal. burned
			low	med	high	
TOTAL CALORIES BURNED						

COMMENTS:

Type:
Qty:
Type:
Qty:
Type:
Qty:
Type:
Qty:
Type:
Qty:
Type:
Qty:

Daily Assessment and Notes

OBSTACLES, SOLUTIONS AND THOUGHTS ON YOUR PROGRESS

Daily Nutritional Intake

FOOD AND BEVERAGES

Eating fish is a
good way to
increase the healthy
fats in your diet,
which can help
reduce the risk of
heart attacks. Fish
is also a great
source of protein,
zinc and iron and
has less saturated
fat, which can
increase blood
cholesterol.

MORNING TIME:	amt.	cal.	fat gms	protein gms	carbs. gms	fiber gms
BREAKFAST TOTALS						

COMMENTS:

AFTERNOON TIME:	amt.	cal.	fat gms	protein gms	carbs. gms	fiber gms
LUNCH TOTALS						

COMMENTS:

Daily Serving Intake

_____ Fruits
# of servings

_____ Vegetables
# of servings

_____ Grains
# of servings

_____ Meat & Beans
# of servings

_____ Milk & Dairy
# of servings

_____ Oils & Sweets
# of servings

EVENING TIME:	amt.	cal.	fat gms	protein gms	carbs. gms	fiber gms
DINNER TOTALS						

COMMENTS:

Water Intake

oz.

118

❏ low ❏ med ❏ high

ENERGY LEVELS

Daily Nutritional Intake

FOOD AND BEVERAGES

DAILY GOALS
ACHIEVED

DAILY TOTALS

SNACKS TIME:	amt.	cal.	fat gms	protein gms	carbs. gms	fiber gms
SNACK TOTALS						

COMMENTS:

Calories

Fat

Protein

Carbohydrates

Fiber

Other

Exercise and Fitness

DAILY PHYSICAL ACTIVITIES

VITAMINS &
SUPPLEMENTS

ACTIVITY/ EXERCISE	hrs./ mins.	reps./ sets	low	med	high	cal. burned
TOTAL CALORIES BURNED						

INTENSITY

COMMENTS:

Type:

Qty:

Type:

Qty:

Type:

Qty:

Type:

Qty:

Type:

Qty:

Type:

Qty:

Daily Assessment and Notes

OBSTACLES, SOLUTIONS AND THOUGHTS ON YOUR PROGRESS

Daily Nutritional Intake

FOOD AND BEVERAGES

Daily Serving Intake

_____ Fruits
# of servings

_____ Vegetables
# of servings

_____ Grains
# of servings

_____ Meat & Beans
# of servings

_____ Milk & Dairy
# of servings

_____ Oils & Sweets
# of servings

Water Intake

oz.

MORNING TIME:	amt.	cal.	fat gms	protein gms	carbs. gms	fiber gms
BREAKFAST TOTALS						

COMMENTS:

AFTERNOON TIME:	amt.	cal.	fat gms	protein gms	carbs. gms	fiber gms
LUNCH TOTALS						

COMMENTS:

EVENING TIME:	amt.	cal.	fat gms	protein gms	carbs. gms	fiber gms
DINNER TOTALS						

COMMENTS:

Daily Nutritional Intake

FOOD AND BEVERAGES

DAILY GOALS
ACHIEVED

DAILY TOTALS

SNACKS TIME:	amt.	cal.	fat gms	protein gms	carbs. gms	fiber gms
SNACK TOTALS						

COMMENTS:

Calories

Fat

Protein

Carbohydrates

Fiber

Other

Exercise and Fitness

DAILY PHYSICAL ACTIVITIES

VITAMINS &
SUPPLEMENTS

ACTIVITY/ EXERCISE	hrs./ mins.	reps./ sets	------INTENSITY------ low	med	high	cal. burned
TOTAL CALORIES BURNED						

COMMENTS:

Type:

Qty:

Type:

Qty:

Type:

Qty:

Type:

Qty:

Type:

Qty:

Type:

Qty:

Daily Assessment and Notes

OBSTACLES, SOLUTIONS AND THOUGHTS ON YOUR PROGRESS

Daily Nutritional Intake

**Helpful Tips
for Effective
Weight-Loss**

Body mass index
(BMI) is a good
way to provide an
idea about your
weight. However,
to get an accurate
assessment of your
health, you need to
include a review of
your physical activity, growth and
muscle mass.

FOOD AND BEVERAGES

MORNING TIME:	amt.	cal.	fat gms	protein gms	carbs. gms	fiber gms
BREAKFAST TOTALS						

COMMENTS:

AFTERNOON TIME:	amt.	cal.	fat gms	protein gms	carbs. gms	fiber gms
LUNCH TOTALS						

COMMENTS:

EVENING TIME:	amt.	cal.	fat gms	protein gms	carbs. gms	fiber gms
DINNER TOTALS						

COMMENTS:

Daily Serving Intake

_____ Fruits
# of servings

_____ Vegetables
# of servings

_____ Grains
# of servings

_____ Meat & Beans
# of servings

_____ Milk & Dairy
# of servings

_____ Oils & Sweets
# of servings

Water Intake

oz.

Daily Nutritional Intake

FOOD AND BEVERAGES

I DID IT!

DAILY GOALS
ACHIEVED

DAILY TOTALS

SNACKS TIME:	amt.	cal.	fat gms	protein gms	carbs. gms	fiber gms
SNACK TOTALS						

COMMENTS:

Calories

Fat

Protein

Carbohydrates

Fiber

Other

Exercise and Fitness

DAILY PHYSICAL ACTIVITIES

VITAMINS &
SUPPLEMENTS

ACTIVITY/ EXERCISE	hrs./ mins.	reps./ sets	------INTENSITY------			cal. burned
			low	med	high	
TOTAL CALORIES BURNED						

COMMENTS:

Type:

Qty:

Type:

Qty:

Type:

Qty:

Type:

Qty:

Type:

Qty:

Type:

Qty:

Daily Assessment and Notes

OBSTACLES, SOLUTIONS AND THOUGHTS ON YOUR PROGRESS

WEIGHT

Daily Nutritional Intake

FOOD AND BEVERAGES

MORNING TIME:	amt.	cal.	fat gms	protein gms	carbs. gms	fiber gms
BREAKFAST TOTALS						

COMMENTS:

AFTERNOON TIME:	amt.	cal.	fat gms	protein gms	carbs. gms	fiber gms
LUNCH TOTALS						

COMMENTS:

Daily Serving Intake

____ Fruits
# of servings

____ Vegetables
# of servings

____ Grains
# of servings

____ Meat & Beans
# of servings

____ Milk & Dairy
# of servings

____ Oils & Sweets
# of servings

EVENING TIME:	amt.	cal.	fat gms	protein gms	carbs. gms	fiber gms
DINNER TOTALS						

Water Intake

oz.

COMMENTS:

I DID IT!

DAILY GOALS ACHIEVED

Daily Nutritional Intake

FOOD AND BEVERAGES

SNACKS TIME:	amt.	cal.	fat gms	protein gms	carbs. gms	fiber gms
SNACK TOTALS						

COMMENTS:

DAILY TOTALS

Calories

Fat

Protein

Carbohydrates

Fiber

Other

Exercise and Fitness

DAILY PHYSICAL ACTIVITIES

ACTIVITY/ EXERCISE	hrs./ mins.	reps./ sets	------INTENSITY------			cal. burned
			low	med	high	
TOTAL CALORIES BURNED						

COMMENTS:

VITAMINS & SUPPLEMENTS

Type:

Qty:

Type:

Qty:

Type:

Qty:

Type:

Qty:

Type:

Qty:

Type:

Qty:

Daily Assessment and Notes

OBSTACLES, SOLUTIONS AND THOUGHTS ON YOUR PROGRESS

Daily Nutritional Intake

FOOD AND BEVERAGES

MORNING TIME:	amt.	cal.	fat gms	protein gms	carbs. gms	fiber gms
BREAKFAST TOTALS						

COMMENTS:

AFTERNOON TIME:	amt.	cal.	fat gms	protein gms	carbs. gms	fiber gms
LUNCH TOTALS						

COMMENTS:

Daily Serving Intake

_____ Fruits
# of servings

_____ Vegetables
# of servings

_____ Grains
# of servings

_____ Meat & Beans
# of servings

_____ Milk & Dairy
# of servings

_____ Oils & Sweets
# of servings

EVENING TIME:	amt.	cal.	fat gms	protein gms	carbs. gms	fiber gms
DINNER TOTALS						

COMMENTS:

Water Intake

oz.

❏ low   ❏ med   ❏ high

ENERGY LEVELS

Daily Nutritional Intake

FOOD AND BEVERAGES

**DAILY GOALS
ACHIEVED**

SNACKS TIME:	amt.	cal.	fat gms	protein gms	carbs. gms	fiber gms
SNACK TOTALS						

COMMENTS:

DAILY TOTALS

Calories

Fat

Protein

Carbohydrates

Fiber

Other

Exercise and Fitness

DAILY PHYSICAL ACTIVITIES

**VITAMINS &
SUPPLEMENTS**

ACTIVITY/ EXERCISE	hrs./ mins.	reps./ sets	low	med	high	cal. burned
TOTAL CALORIES BURNED						

------INTENSITY------

COMMENTS:

Type:

Qty:

Type:

Qty:

Type:

Qty:

Type:

Qty:

Type:

Qty:

Type:

Qty:

Daily Assessment and Notes

OBSTACLES, SOLUTIONS AND THOUGHTS ON YOUR PROGRESS

Helpful Tips for Effective Weight-Loss

Ever wonder the difference between "enriched" foods and "fortified" foods?

Enriched foods have nutrients added to them that were lost during food processing. Fortified foods have nutrients added that were not originally present.

Daily Serving Intake

_____ Fruits
# of servings

_____ Vegetables
# of servings

_____ Grains
# of servings

_____ Meat & Beans
# of servings

_____ Milk & Dairy
# of servings

_____ Oils & Sweets
# of servings

Water Intake

oz. _____

Daily Nutritional Intake

FOOD AND BEVERAGES

MORNING TIME:	amt.	cal.	fat gms	protein gms	carbs. gms	fiber gms
BREAKFAST TOTALS						

COMMENTS:

AFTERNOON TIME:	amt.	cal.	fat gms	protein gms	carbs. gms	fiber gms
LUNCH TOTALS						

COMMENTS:

EVENING TIME:	amt.	cal.	fat gms	protein gms	carbs. gms	fiber gms
DINNER TOTALS						

COMMENTS:

☐ low ☐ med ☐ high

ENERGY LEVELS

Daily Nutritional Intake

FOOD AND BEVERAGES

SNACKS TIME:	amt.	cal.	fat gms	protein gms	carbs. gms	fiber gms
SNACK TOTALS						

COMMENTS:

DAILY TOTALS

Calories

Fat

Protein

Carbohydrates

Fiber

Other

Exercise and Fitness

DAILY PHYSICAL ACTIVITIES

ACTIVITY/ EXERCISE	hrs./ mins.	reps./ sets	------INTENSITY------			cal. burned
			low	med	high	
TOTAL CALORIES BURNED						

COMMENTS:

VITAMINS &
SUPPLEMENTS

Type:

Qty:

Type:

Qty:

Type:

Qty:

Type:

Qty:

Type:

Qty:

Type:

Qty:

Daily Assessment and Notes

OBSTACLES, SOLUTIONS AND THOUGHTS ON YOUR PROGRESS

Daily Nutritional Intake

FOOD AND BEVERAGES

Helpful Tips
for Effective
Weight-Loss

Eating 5 small
meals a day is a
good way to
control your eating
habits, portion
sizes, and help you
lose weight. By
eating 5 smaller
meals, you will
never feel deprived
and risk going off
your weight-loss
program.

MORNING TIME:		amt.	cal.	fat gms	protein gms	carbs. gms	fiber gms
BREAKFAST TOTALS							

COMMENTS:

AFTERNOON TIME:		amt.	cal.	fat gms	protein gms	carbs. gms	fiber gms
LUNCH TOTALS							

COMMENTS:

Daily Serving Intake

____ Fruits
# of servings

____ Vegetables
# of servings

____ Grains
# of servings

____ Meat & Beans
# of servings

____ Milk & Dairy
# of servings

____ Oils & Sweets
# of servings

EVENING TIME:		amt.	cal.	fat gms	protein gms	carbs. gms	fiber gms
DINNER TOTALS							

Water Intake

oz.

COMMENTS:

130

❏ low ❏ med ❏ high

ENERGY LEVELS

Daily Nutritional Intake

FOOD AND BEVERAGES

DAILY TOTALS

SNACKS TIME:	amt.	cal.	fat gms	protein gms	carbs. gms	fiber gms
SNACK TOTALS						

COMMENTS:

Calories

Fat

Protein

Carbohydrates

Fiber

Other

Exercise and Fitness

DAILY PHYSICAL ACTIVITIES

VITAMINS &
SUPPLEMENTS

ACTIVITY/ EXERCISE	hrs./ mins.	reps./ sets	------INTENSITY------ low	med	high	cal. burned
TOTAL CALORIES BURNED						

COMMENTS:

Type:
Qty:
Type:
Qty:
Type:
Qty:
Type:
Qty:
Type:
Qty:
Type:
Qty:

Daily Assessment and Notes

OBSTACLES, SOLUTIONS AND THOUGHTS ON YOUR PROGRESS

Daily Nutritional Intake

FOOD AND BEVERAGES

If you have a sweet tooth, take heart! The sweetness you crave can often be achieved by adding spices to bring out the flavor of certain foods.

Ginger, cinnamon, nutmeg, and vanilla are all good ways to enhance the flavor of foods that otherwise may not have been considered sweet.

MORNING TIME:	amt.	cal.	fat gms	protein gms	carbs. gms	fiber gms
BREAKFAST TOTALS						

COMMENTS:

AFTERNOON TIME:	amt.	cal.	fat gms	protein gms	carbs. gms	fiber gms
LUNCH TOTALS						

COMMENTS:

Daily Serving Intake

_____ Fruits
# of servings

_____ Vegetables
# of servings

_____ Grains
# of servings

_____ Meat & Beans
# of servings

_____ Milk & Dairy
# of servings

_____ Oils & Sweets
# of servings

EVENING TIME:	amt.	cal.	fat gms	protein gms	carbs. gms	fiber gms
DINNER TOTALS						

Water Intake

oz.

COMMENTS:

132

❏ low ❏ med ❏ high

ENERGY LEVELS

Daily Nutritional Intake
FOOD AND BEVERAGES

DAILY TOTALS

SNACKS TIME:	amt.	cal.	fat gms	protein gms	carbs. gms	fiber gms
SNACK TOTALS						

COMMENTS:

Calories

Fat

Protein

Carbohydrates

Fiber

Other

Exercise and Fitness
DAILY PHYSICAL ACTIVITIES

VITAMINS &
SUPPLEMENTS

ACTIVITY/ EXERCISE	hrs./ mins.	reps./ sets	low	med	high	cal. burned
			------INTENSITY------			
TOTAL CALORIES BURNED						

COMMENTS:

Type:
Qty:
Type:
Qty:
Type:
Qty:
Type:
Qty:
Type:
Qty:
Type:
Qty:

Daily Assessment and Notes
OBSTACLES, SOLUTIONS AND THOUGHTS ON YOUR PROGRESS

Helpful Tips
for Effective
Weight-Loss

If you're looking
for a quick after-
noon snack, but
want to avoid the
vending machine,
try munching on
slices of fruit, low-
fat popcorn, mixed
nuts or trail mix.
They are healthy
alternatives to the
candy and chips
often found in
vending machines.

Daily Nutritional Intake

FOOD AND BEVERAGES

MORNING TIME:	amt.	cal.	fat gms	protein gms	carbs. gms	fiber gms
BREAKFAST TOTALS						

COMMENTS:

AFTERNOON TIME:	amt.	cal.	fat gms	protein gms	carbs. gms	fiber gms
LUNCH TOTALS						

COMMENTS:

EVENING TIME:	amt.	cal.	fat gms	protein gms	carbs. gms	fiber gms
DINNER TOTALS						

COMMENTS:

Daily Serving Intake

____ Fruits
# of servings

____ Vegetables
# of servings

____ Grains
# of servings

____ Meat & Beans
# of servings

____ Milk & Dairy
# of servings

____ Oils & Sweets
# of servings

Water Intake

oz. ____

◻ low ◻ med ◻ high

ENERGY LEVELS

Daily Nutritional Intake

FOOD AND BEVERAGES

I DID IT!

DAILY GOALS
ACHIEVED

SNACKS TIME:	amt.	cal.	fat gms	protein gms	carbs. gms	fiber gms
SNACK TOTALS						

COMMENTS:

DAILY TOTALS

Calories

Fat

Protein

Carbohydrates

Fiber

Other

Exercise and Fitness

DAILY PHYSICAL ACTIVITIES

ACTIVITY/ EXERCISE	hrs./ mins.	reps./ sets	------INTENSITY------ low	med	high	cal. burned
TOTAL CALORIES BURNED						

COMMENTS:

VITAMINS &
SUPPLEMENTS

Type:

Qty:

Type:

Qty:

Type:

Qty:

Type:

Qty:

Type:

Qty:

Type:

Qty:

Daily Assessment and Notes

OBSTACLES, SOLUTIONS AND THOUGHTS ON YOUR PROGRESS

DATE

WEIGHT

Helpful Tips
for Effective
Weight-Loss

Trans fats occur
as a result of the
hydrogenation
process, which
turns oil into a
more solid fat.
Research shows
that trans fats
increase the LDL,
or "bad" choles-
terol, increasing the
risk of heart
disease.

Beware of trans fats
found in certain
snacks and fried
foods.

Daily Serving Intake

_____ Fruits
# of servings

_____ Vegetables
# of servings

_____ Grains
# of servings

_____ Meat & Beans
# of servings

_____ Milk & Dairy
# of servings

_____ Oils & Sweets
# of servings

Water Intake

oz.

136

Daily Nutritional Intake

FOOD AND BEVERAGES

MORNING TIME:		amt.	cal.	fat gms	protein gms	carbs. gms	fiber gms
BREAKFAST TOTALS							

COMMENTS:

AFTERNOON TIME:		amt.	cal.	fat gms	protein gms	carbs. gms	fiber gms
LUNCH TOTALS							

COMMENTS:

EVENING TIME:		amt.	cal.	fat gms	protein gms	carbs. gms	fiber gms
DINNER TOTALS							

COMMENTS:

DAILY GOALS
ACHIEVED

Daily Nutritional Intake

FOOD AND BEVERAGES

DAILY TOTALS

SNACKS TIME:	amt.	cal.	fat gms	protein gms	carbs. gms	fiber gms
SNACK TOTALS						

COMMENTS:

Calories

Fat

Protein

Carbohydrates

Fiber

Other

Exercise and Fitness

DAILY PHYSICAL ACTIVITIES

VITAMINS &
SUPPLEMENTS

ACTIVITY/ EXERCISE	hrs./ mins.	reps./ sets	------INTENSITY------ low	med	high	cal. burned
TOTAL CALORIES BURNED						

COMMENTS:

Type:
Qty:
Type:
Qty:
Type:
Qty:
Type:
Qty:
Type:
Qty:
Type:
Qty:

Daily Assessment and Notes

OBSTACLES, SOLUTIONS AND THOUGHTS ON YOUR PROGRESS

WEIGHT

Daily Nutritional Intake

FOOD AND BEVERAGES

When eating, try to
savor each bite of
food, while putting
your fork down
between bites. This
can help you con-
trol your portion
sizes so you don't
overeat.

MORNING TIME:		amt.	cal.	fat gms	protein gms	carbs. gms	fiber gms
BREAKFAST TOTALS							

COMMENTS:

AFTERNOON TIME:		amt.	cal.	fat gms	protein gms	carbs. gms	fiber gms
LUNCH TOTALS							

COMMENTS:

Daily Serving Intake

_____ Fruits
# of servings

_____ Vegetables
# of servings

_____ Grains
# of servings

_____ Meat & Beans
# of servings

_____ Milk & Dairy
# of servings

_____ Oils & Sweets
# of servings

Water Intake

oz. _____

EVENING TIME:		amt.	cal.	fat gms	protein gms	carbs. gms	fiber gms
DINNER TOTALS							

COMMENTS:

I DID IT!

DAILY GOALS
ACHIEVED

Daily Nutritional Intake

FOOD AND BEVERAGES

DAILY TOTALS

SNACKS TIME:	amt.	cal.	fat gms	protein gms	carbs. gms	fiber gms
SNACK TOTALS						

COMMENTS:

Calories

Fat

Protein

Carbohydrates

Fiber

Other

Exercise and Fitness

DAILY PHYSICAL ACTIVITIES

VITAMINS & SUPPLEMENTS

ACTIVITY/ EXERCISE	hrs./ mins.	reps./ sets	low	med	high	cal. burned
TOTAL CALORIES BURNED						

INTENSITY

COMMENTS:

Type:

Qty:

Type:

Qty:

Type:

Qty:

Type:

Qty:

Type:

Qty:

Type:

Qty:

Daily Assessment and Notes

OBSTACLES, SOLUTIONS AND THOUGHTS ON YOUR PROGRESS

DATE _____   WEIGHT _____

Helpful Tips
for Effective
Weight-Loss

Men and women
who eat breakfast
in the mornings are
far less likely to
become obese than
those who skip the
most important
meal of the day.

Start with a healthy
meal, and you will
be more likely to
continue those
healthy eating
habits throughout
the day.

Daily Serving Intake

_____ Fruits
        # of servings

_____ Vegetables
        # of servings

_____ Grains
        # of servings

_____ Meat & Beans
        # of servings

_____ Milk & Dairy
        # of servings

_____ Oils & Sweets
        # of servings

Water Intake

oz. _____

140

Daily Nutritional Intake

FOOD AND BEVERAGES

MORNING TIME:	amt.	cal.	fat gms	protein gms	carbs. gms	fiber gms
BREAKFAST TOTALS						

COMMENTS:

AFTERNOON TIME:	amt.	cal.	fat gms	protein gms	carbs. gms	fiber gms
LUNCH TOTALS						

COMMENTS:

EVENING TIME:	amt.	cal.	fat gms	protein gms	carbs. gms	fiber gms
DINNER TOTALS						

COMMENTS:

❏ low   ❏ med   ❏ high

ENERGY LEVELS

Daily Nutritional Intake

FOOD AND BEVERAGES

**DAILY GOALS
ACHIEVED**

SNACKS TIME:	amt.	cal.	fat gms	protein gms	carbs. gms	fiber gms
SNACK TOTALS						

COMMENTS:

DAILY TOTALS

Calories

Fat

Protein

Carbohydrates

Fiber

Other

Exercise and Fitness

DAILY PHYSICAL ACTIVITIES

**VITAMINS &
SUPPLEMENTS**

ACTIVITY/ EXERCISE	hrs./ mins.	reps./ sets	------INTENSITY------ low	med	high	cal. burned
TOTAL CALORIES BURNED						

COMMENTS:

Type:

Qty:

Type:

Qty:

Type:

Qty:

Type:

Qty:

Type:

Qty:

Type:

Qty:

Daily Assessment and Notes

OBSTACLES, SOLUTIONS AND THOUGHTS ON YOUR PROGRESS

DATE   WEIGHT

Helpful Tips
for Effective
Weight-Loss

Try not to go to the
grocery store when
you are hungry. It
can lead you to buy
more food than you
need, or foods that
don't normally fit
into your weight-
loss program.

Daily Nutritional Intake

FOOD AND BEVERAGES

MORNING TIME:	amt.	cal.	fat gms	protein gms	carbs. gms	fiber gms
BREAKFAST TOTALS						

COMMENTS:

AFTERNOON TIME:	amt.	cal.	fat gms	protein gms	carbs. gms	fiber gms
LUNCH TOTALS						

COMMENTS:

EVENING TIME:	amt.	cal.	fat gms	protein gms	carbs. gms	fiber gms
DINNER TOTALS						

COMMENTS:

Daily Serving Intake

_____ Fruits
      # of servings

_____ Vegetables
      # of servings

_____ Grains
      # of servings

_____ Meat & Beans
      # of servings

_____ Milk & Dairy
      # of servings

_____ Oils & Sweets
      # of servings

Water Intake

oz.

142

☐ low ☐ med ☐ high

ENERGY LEVELS

Daily Nutritional Intake

FOOD AND BEVERAGES

**DAILY GOALS
ACHIEVED**

DAILY TOTALS

SNACKS TIME:	amt.	cal.	fat gms	protein gms	carbs. gms	fiber gms
SNACK TOTALS						

COMMENTS:

Calories

Fat

Protein

Carbohydrates

Fiber

Other

Exercise and Fitness

DAILY PHYSICAL ACTIVITIES

**VITAMINS &
SUPPLEMENTS**

ACTIVITY/ EXERCISE	hrs./ mins.	reps./ sets	-----INTENSITY----- low	med	high	cal. burned
TOTAL CALORIES BURNED						

COMMENTS:

Type:

Qty:

Type:

Qty:

Type:

Qty:

Type:

Qty:

Type:

Qty:

Type:

Qty:

Daily Assessment and Notes

OBSTACLES, SOLUTIONS AND THOUGHTS ON YOUR PROGRESS

DATE _____   WEIGHT _____

**Helpful Tips
for Effective
Weight-Loss**

Nuts are a great
snack item.
They are high in
monounsaturated
fats, protein, carbo-
hydrates, as well as
vitamins and
minerals.

Snacking on nuts
can help lead you
to eat less and lose
weight. However,
since nuts are high
in calories, just be
sure to eat only
small servings at a
time.

Daily Nutritional Intake

FOOD AND BEVERAGES

MORNING TIME:	amt.	cal.	fat gms	protein gms	carbs. gms	fiber gms
BREAKFAST TOTALS						

COMMENTS:

AFTERNOON TIME:	amt.	cal.	fat gms	protein gms	carbs. gms	fiber gms
LUNCH TOTALS						

COMMENTS:

Daily Serving Intake

____ Fruits
      # of servings

____ Vegetables
      # of servings

____ Grains
      # of servings

____ Meat & Beans
      # of servings

____ Milk & Dairy
      # of servings

____ Oils & Sweets
      # of servings

Water Intake

oz. _____

EVENING TIME:	amt.	cal.	fat gms	protein gms	carbs. gms	fiber gms
DINNER TOTALS						

COMMENTS:

I DID IT!

DAILY GOALS
ACHIEVED

Daily Nutritional Intake

FOOD AND BEVERAGES

DAILY TOTALS

SNACKS TIME:	amt.	cal.	fat gms	protein gms	carbs. gms	fiber gms
SNACK TOTALS						

COMMENTS:

Calories

Fat

Protein

Carbohydrates

Fiber

Other

Exercise and Fitness

DAILY PHYSICAL ACTIVITIES

VITAMINS &
SUPPLEMENTS

ACTIVITY/ EXERCISE	hrs./ mins.	reps./ sets	INTENSITY low	med	high	cal. burned
TOTAL CALORIES BURNED						

COMMENTS:

Type:

Qty:

Type:

Qty:

Type:

Qty:

Type:

Qty:

Type:

Qty:

Type:

Qty:

Daily Assessment and Notes

OBSTACLES, SOLUTIONS AND THOUGHTS ON YOUR PROGRESS

WEIGHT

Daily Nutritional Intake

FOOD AND BEVERAGES

MORNING TIME:	amt.	cal.	fat gms	protein gms	carbs. gms	fiber gms
BREAKFAST TOTALS						

COMMENTS:

AFTERNOON TIME:	amt.	cal.	fat gms	protein gms	carbs. gms	fiber gms
LUNCH TOTALS						

COMMENTS:

EVENING TIME:	amt.	cal.	fat gms	protein gms	carbs. gms	fiber gms
DINNER TOTALS						

COMMENTS:

Daily Serving Intake

_____ Fruits
# of servings

_____ Vegetables
# of servings

_____ Grains
# of servings

_____ Meat & Beans
# of servings

_____ Milk & Dairy
# of servings

_____ Oils & Sweets
# of servings

Water Intake

oz. _____

low ☐ med ☐ high

ENERGY LEVELS

Daily Nutritional Intake

FOOD AND BEVERAGES

DAILY TOTALS

SNACKS TIME:	amt.	cal.	fat gms	protein gms	carbs. gms	fiber gms
SNACK TOTALS						

COMMENTS:

Calories

Fat

Protein

Carbohydrates

Fiber

Other

Exercise and Fitness

DAILY PHYSICAL ACTIVITIES

VITAMINS &
SUPPLEMENTS

ACTIVITY/ EXERCISE	hrs./ mins.	reps./ sets	------INTENSITY------			cal. burned
			low	med	high	
TOTAL CALORIES BURNED						

COMMENTS:

Type:

Qty:

Type:

Qty:

Type:

Qty:

Type:

Qty:

Type:

Qty:

Type:

Qty:

Daily Assessment and Notes

OBSTACLES, SOLUTIONS AND THOUGHTS ON YOUR PROGRESS

Daily Nutritional Intake

**Helpful Tips
for Effective
Weight-Loss**

Try grilling,
sautéing, or baking
your food instead
of frying. The way
you prepare your
food is important
to lead to a healthi-
er lifestyle and
weight-loss.

Daily Serving Intake

____ Fruits
# of servings

____ Vegetables
# of servings

____ Grains
# of servings

____ Meat & Beans
# of servings

____ Milk & Dairy
# of servings

____ Oils & Sweets
# of servings

Water Intake

oz. _____

FOOD AND BEVERAGES

MORNING TIME:	amt.	cal.	fat gms	protein gms	carbs. gms	fiber gms
BREAKFAST TOTALS						

COMMENTS:

AFTERNOON TIME:	amt.	cal.	fat gms	protein gms	carbs. gms	fiber gms
LUNCH TOTALS						

COMMENTS:

EVENING TIME:	amt.	cal.	fat gms	protein gms	carbs. gms	fiber gms
DINNER TOTALS						

COMMENTS:

148

☐ low ☐ med ☐ high

ENERGY LEVELS

Daily Nutritional Intake

FOOD AND BEVERAGES

DAILY GOALS
ACHIEVED

SNACKS TIME:	amt.	cal.	fat gms	protein gms	carbs. gms	fiber gms
SNACK TOTALS						

COMMENTS:

DAILY TOTALS

Calories

Fat

Protein

Carbohydrates

Fiber

Other

Exercise and Fitness

DAILY PHYSICAL ACTIVITIES

VITAMINS &
SUPPLEMENTS

ACTIVITY/ EXERCISE	hrs./ mins.	reps./ sets	------INTENSITY------			cal. burned
			low	med	high	
TOTAL CALORIES BURNED						

COMMENTS:

Type:

Qty:

Type:

Qty:

Type:

Qty:

Type:

Qty:

Type:

Qty:

Type:

Qty:

Daily Assessment and Notes

OBSTACLES, SOLUTIONS AND THOUGHTS ON YOUR PROGRESS

Helpful Tips
for Effective
Weight-Loss

Daily Nutritional Intake

FOOD AND BEVERAGES

When eating a
sandwich, try to
choose whole grain
bread over white
bread or a wrap.
Whole grain bread
provides you with
more fiber and
other healthy
nutrients.

MORNING TIME:	amt.	cal.	fat gms	protein gms	carbs. gms	fiber gms
BREAKFAST TOTALS						

COMMENTS:

AFTERNOON TIME:	amt.	cal.	fat gms	protein gms	carbs. gms	fiber gms
LUNCH TOTALS						

COMMENTS:

Daily Serving Intake

____ Fruits
     # of servings

____ Vegetables
     # of servings

____ Grains
     # of servings

____ Meat & Beans
     # of servings

____ Milk & Dairy
     # of servings

____ Oils & Sweets
     # of servings

EVENING TIME:	amt.	cal.	fat gms	protein gms	carbs. gms	fiber gms
DINNER TOTALS						

COMMENTS:

Water Intake

oz.

ENERGY LEVELS

Daily Nutritional Intake

FOOD AND BEVERAGES

**DAILY GOALS
ACHIEVED**

DAILY TOTALS

SNACKS TIME:	amt.	cal.	fat gms	protein gms	carbs. gms	fiber gms
SNACK TOTALS						

COMMENTS:

Calories

Fat

Protein

Carbohydrates

Fiber

Other

Exercise and Fitness

DAILY PHYSICAL ACTIVITIES

**VITAMINS &
SUPPLEMENTS**

ACTIVITY/ EXERCISE	hrs./ mins.	reps./ sets	------INTENSITY------ low	med	high	cal. burned
TOTAL CALORIES BURNED						

COMMENTS:

Type:
Qty:
Type:
Qty:
Type:
Qty:
Type:
Qty:
Type:
Qty:
Type:
Qty:

Daily Assessment and Notes

OBSTACLES, SOLUTIONS AND THOUGHTS ON YOUR PROGRESS

Daily Nutritional Intake

FOOD AND BEVERAGES

If you feel a
craving, but do not
want to go off your
weight-loss
program, try to
distract yourself by
taking a walk or
calling a friend.
The craving will
pass within a few
moments.

MORNING TIME:	amt.	cal.	fat gms	protein gms	carbs. gms	fiber gms
BREAKFAST TOTALS						

COMMENTS:

AFTERNOON TIME:	amt.	cal.	fat gms	protein gms	carbs. gms	fiber gms
LUNCH TOTALS						

COMMENTS:

Daily Serving Intake

____ Fruits
# of servings

____ Vegetables
# of servings

____ Grains
# of servings

____ Meat & Beans
# of servings

____ Milk & Dairy
# of servings

____ Oils & Sweets
# of servings

Water Intake

oz.

EVENING TIME:	amt.	cal.	fat gms	protein gms	carbs. gms	fiber gms
DINNER TOTALS						

COMMENTS:

❑ low ❑ med ❑ high

ENERGY LEVELS

Daily Nutritional Intake

FOOD AND BEVERAGES

**DAILY GOALS
ACHIEVED**

SNACKS TIME:	amt.	cal.	fat gms	protein gms	carbs. gms	fiber gms
SNACK TOTALS						

COMMENTS:

DAILY TOTALS

Calories

Fat

Protein

Carbohydrates

Fiber

Other

Exercise and Fitness

DAILY PHYSICAL ACTIVITIES

ACTIVITY/ EXERCISE	hrs./ mins.	reps./ sets	------INTENSITY------ low	med	high	cal. burned
TOTAL CALORIES BURNED						

COMMENTS:

**VITAMINS &
SUPPLEMENTS**

Type:

Qty:

Type:

Qty:

Type:

Qty:

Type:

Qty:

Type:

Qty:

Type:

Qty:

Daily Assessment and Notes

OBSTACLES, SOLUTIONS AND THOUGHTS ON YOUR PROGRESS

Daily Nutritional Intake

FOOD AND BEVERAGES

Helpful Tips
for Effective
Weight-Loss

Keep healthy
snacks in your
kitchen. That way,
when you have the
urge to munch on
something, you will
have better choices
on hand.

MORNING TIME:	amt.	cal.	fat gms	protein gms	carbs. gms	fiber gms
BREAKFAST TOTALS						

COMMENTS:

AFTERNOON TIME:	amt.	cal.	fat gms	protein gms	carbs. gms	fiber gms
LUNCH TOTALS						

COMMENTS:

Daily Serving Intake

_____ Fruits
# of servings

_____ Vegetables
# of servings

_____ Grains
# of servings

_____ Meat & Beans
# of servings

_____ Milk & Dairy
# of servings

_____ Oils & Sweets
# of servings

EVENING TIME:	amt.	cal.	fat gms	protein gms	carbs. gms	fiber gms
DINNER TOTALS						

Water Intake

oz. _____

COMMENTS:

❑ low   ❑ med   ❑ high

ENERGY LEVELS

Daily Nutritional Intake

FOOD AND BEVERAGES

DAILY TOTALS

SNACKS TIME:	amt.	cal.	fat gms	protein gms	carbs. gms	fiber gms
SNACK TOTALS						

COMMENTS:

Calories

Fat

Protein

Carbohydrates

Fiber

Other

Exercise and Fitness

DAILY PHYSICAL ACTIVITIES

VITAMINS &
SUPPLEMENTS

ACTIVITY/ EXERCISE	hrs./ mins.	reps./ sets	------INTENSITY------			cal. burned
			low	med	high	
TOTAL CALORIES BURNED						

COMMENTS:

Type:
Qty:
Type:
Qty:
Type:
Qty:
Type:
Qty:
Type:
Qty:
Type:
Qty:

Daily Assessment and Notes

OBSTACLES, SOLUTIONS AND THOUGHTS ON YOUR PROGRESS

Tips for
healthy
living

Daily Nutritional Intake

FOOD AND BEVERAGES

Even if you are
cutting back on fat,
it is still important
to include some
form of this vital
nutrient into your
diet.

Just make sure that
the fat you do con-
sume is the healthy,
unsaturated kind
found in fish, nuts
and seeds.

MORNING TIME:	amt.	cal.	fat gms	protein gms	carbs. gms	fiber gms
BREAKFAST TOTALS						

COMMENTS:

AFTERNOON TIME:	amt.	cal.	fat gms	protein gms	carbs. gms	fiber gms
LUNCH TOTALS						

COMMENTS:

Daily Serving Intake

_____ Fruits
# of servings

_____ Vegetables
# of servings

_____ Grains
# of servings

_____ Meat & Beans
# of servings

_____ Milk & Dairy
# of servings

_____ Oils & Sweets
# of servings

Water Intake

oz. _____

EVENING TIME:	amt.	cal.	fat gms	protein gms	carbs. gms	fiber gms
DINNER TOTALS						

COMMENTS:

❏ low ❏ med ❏ high

ENERGY LEVELS

Daily Nutritional Intake
FOOD AND BEVERAGES

DAILY GOALS ACHIEVED

DAILY TOTALS

SNACKS TIME:	amt.	cal.	fat gms	protein gms	carbs. gms	fiber gms
SNACK TOTALS						

COMMENTS:

Calories

Fat

Protein

Carbohydrates

Fiber

Other

Exercise and Fitness
DAILY PHYSICAL ACTIVITIES

VITAMINS & SUPPLEMENTS

ACTIVITY/ EXERCISE	hrs./ mins.	reps./ sets	low	med	high	cal. burned
TOTAL CALORIES BURNED						

Table header: ------INTENSITY------ (spanning low, med, high)

COMMENTS:

Type:
Qty:
Type:
Qty:
Type:
Qty:
Type:
Qty:
Type:
Qty:
Type:
Qty:

Daily Assessment and Notes
OBSTACLES, SOLUTIONS AND THOUGHTS ON YOUR PROGRESS

Daily Nutritional Intake

FOOD AND BEVERAGES

MORNING TIME:	amt.	cal.	fat gms	protein gms	carbs. gms	fiber gms
BREAKFAST TOTALS						

COMMENTS:

AFTERNOON TIME:	amt.	cal.	fat gms	protein gms	carbs. gms	fiber gms
LUNCH TOTALS						

COMMENTS:

Daily Serving Intake

____ Fruits
      # of servings

____ Vegetables
      # of servings

____ Grains
      # of servings

____ Meat & Beans
      # of servings

____ Milk & Dairy
      # of servings

____ Oils & Sweets
      # of servings

EVENING TIME:	amt.	cal.	fat gms	protein gms	carbs. gms	fiber gms
DINNER TOTALS						

Water Intake

COMMENTS:

oz.

☐ low ☐ med ☐ high

ENERGY LEVELS

**DAILY GOALS
ACHIEVED**

Daily Nutritional Intake

FOOD AND BEVERAGES

DAILY TOTALS

SNACKS TIME:	amt.	cal.	fat gms	protein gms	carbs. gms	fiber gms
SNACK TOTALS						

COMMENTS:

Calories

Fat

Protein

Carbohydrates

Fiber

Other

Exercise and Fitness

DAILY PHYSICAL ACTIVITIES

**VITAMINS &
SUPPLEMENTS**

ACTIVITY/ EXERCISE	hrs./ mins.	reps./ sets	------INTENSITY------			cal. burned
			low	med	high	
TOTAL CALORIES BURNED						

COMMENTS:

Type:
Qty:
Type:
Qty:
Type:
Qty:
Type:
Qty:
Type:
Qty:
Type:
Qty:

Daily Assessment and Notes

OBSTACLES, SOLUTIONS AND THOUGHTS ON YOUR PROGRESS

**Helpful Tips
for Effective
Weight-Loss**

Daily Nutritional Intake

FOOD AND BEVERAGES

MORNING TIME:	amt.	cal.	fat gms	protein gms	carbs. gms	fiber gms
BREAKFAST TOTALS						

COMMENTS:

If you are headed
to a party where
hors d'oeuvres and
bowls of snacks
will be served, try
to eat a small meal
beforehand, so you
can avoid overeat-
ing or munching on
all the snacks when
you arrive.

AFTERNOON TIME:	amt.	cal.	fat gms	protein gms	carbs. gms	fiber gms
LUNCH TOTALS						

COMMENTS:

Daily Serving Intake

_____ Fruits
    # of servings

_____ Vegetables
    # of servings

_____ Grains
    # of servings

EVENING TIME:	amt.	cal.	fat gms	protein gms	carbs. gms	fiber gms
DINNER TOTALS						

COMMENTS:

_____ Meat & Beans
    # of servings

_____ Milk & Dairy
    # of servings

_____ Oils & Sweets
    # of servings

Water Intake

oz. _____

❑ low   ❑ med   ❑ high

ENERGY LEVELS

Daily Nutritional Intake

FOOD AND BEVERAGES

DAILY TOTALS

SNACKS TIME:	amt.	cal.	fat gms	protein gms	carbs. gms	fiber gms
SNACK TOTALS						

COMMENTS:

Calories

Fat

Protein

Carbohydrates

Fiber

Other

Exercise and Fitness

DAILY PHYSICAL ACTIVITIES

VITAMINS &

SUPPLEMENTS

ACTIVITY/ EXERCISE	hrs./ mins.	reps./ sets	------INTENSITY------ low	med	high	cal. burned
TOTAL CALORIES BURNED						

COMMENTS:

Type:

Qty:

Type:

Qty:

Type:

Qty:

Type:

Qty:

Type:

Qty:

Type:

Qty:

Daily Assessment and Notes

OBSTACLES, SOLUTIONS AND THOUGHTS ON YOUR PROGRESS

Daily Nutritional Intake

FOOD AND BEVERAGES

MORNING TIME:	amt.	cal.	fat gms	protein gms	carbs. gms	fiber gms
BREAKFAST TOTALS						

COMMENTS:

AFTERNOON TIME:	amt.	cal.	fat gms	protein gms	carbs. gms	fiber gms
LUNCH TOTALS						

COMMENTS:

Daily Serving Intake

_____ Fruits
# of servings

_____ Vegetables
# of servings

_____ Grains
# of servings

_____ Meat & Beans
# of servings

_____ Milk & Dairy
# of servings

_____ Oils & Sweets
# of servings

EVENING TIME:	amt.	cal.	fat gms	protein gms	carbs. gms	fiber gms
DINNER TOTALS						

COMMENTS:

Water Intake

oz. _____

❏ low   ❏ med   ❏ high

ENERGY LEVELS

Daily Nutritional Intake

FOOD AND BEVERAGES

**DAILY GOALS
ACHIEVED**

DAILY TOTALS

SNACKS TIME:	amt.	cal.	fat gms	protein gms	carbs. gms	fiber gms
SNACK TOTALS						

COMMENTS:

Calories

Fat

Protein

Carbohydrates

Fiber

Other

Exercise and Fitness

DAILY PHYSICAL ACTIVITIES

**VITAMINS &
SUPPLEMENTS**

ACTIVITY/ EXERCISE	hrs./ mins.	reps./ sets	------INTENSITY------			cal. burned
			low	med	high	
TOTAL CALORIES BURNED						

COMMENTS:

Type:
Qty:
Type:
Qty:
Type:
Qty:
Type:
Qty:
Type:
Qty:
Type:
Qty:
Type:
Qty:

Daily Assessment and Notes

OBSTACLES, SOLUTIONS AND THOUGHTS ON YOUR PROGRESS

Helpful Tips for Effective Weight-Loss

The National Weight Control Registry reports that those who are most successful in losing weight and keeping it off work out regularly, control their calorie intake, and monitor their weight, focusing on smaller portions and healthier food choices.

Daily Nutritional Intake

FOOD AND BEVERAGES

MORNING TIME:	amt.	cal.	fat gms	protein gms	carbs. gms	fiber gms
BREAKFAST TOTALS						

COMMENTS:

AFTERNOON TIME:	amt.	cal.	fat gms	protein gms	carbs. gms	fiber gms
LUNCH TOTALS						

COMMENTS:

EVENING TIME:	amt.	cal.	fat gms	protein gms	carbs. gms	fiber gms
DINNER TOTALS						

COMMENTS:

Daily Serving Intake

_____ Fruits
# of servings

_____ Vegetables
# of servings

_____ Grains
# of servings

_____ Meat & Beans
# of servings

_____ Milk & Dairy
# of servings

_____ Oils & Sweets
# of servings

Water Intake

oz.

❏ low ❏ med ❏ high

ENERGY LEVELS

Daily Nutritional Intake

FOOD AND BEVERAGES

SNACKS TIME:	amt.	cal.	fat gms	protein gms	carbs. gms	fiber gms
SNACK TOTALS						

COMMENTS:

DAILY TOTALS

Calories

Fat

Protein

Carbohydrates

Fiber

Other

Exercise and Fitness

DAILY PHYSICAL ACTIVITIES

ACTIVITY/ EXERCISE	hrs./ mins.	reps./ sets	------INTENSITY------			cal. burned
			low	med	high	
TOTAL CALORIES BURNED						

COMMENTS:

VITAMINS & SUPPLEMENTS

Type:

Qty:

Type:

Qty:

Type:

Qty:

Type:

Qty:

Type:

Qty:

Type:

Qty:

Daily Assessment and Notes

OBSTACLES, SOLUTIONS AND THOUGHTS ON YOUR PROGRESS

WEIGHT

Daily Nutritional Intake

FOOD AND BEVERAGES

Eating a salad
before the start of
your meal can help
curb your appetite,
allowing you to eat
smaller portions of
your main course.

MORNING TIME:	amt.	cal.	fat gms	protein gms	carbs. gms	fiber gms
BREAKFAST TOTALS						

COMMENTS:

AFTERNOON TIME:	amt.	cal.	fat gms	protein gms	carbs. gms	fiber gms
LUNCH TOTALS						

COMMENTS:

Daily Serving Intake

_____ Fruits
# of servings

_____ Vegetables
# of servings

_____ Grains
# of servings

_____ Meat & Beans
# of servings

_____ Milk & Dairy
# of servings

_____ Oils & Sweets
# of servings

EVENING TIME:	amt.	cal.	fat gms	protein gms	carbs. gms	fiber gms
DINNER TOTALS						

Water Intake

oz.

COMMENTS:

❏ low ❏ med ❏ high
ENERGY LEVELS

Daily Nutritional Intake

FOOD AND BEVERAGES

**DAILY GOALS
ACHIEVED**

SNACKS TIME:	amt.	cal.	fat gms	protein gms	carbs. gms	fiber gms
SNACK TOTALS						

COMMENTS:

DAILY TOTALS

Calories

Fat

Protein

Carbohydrates

Fiber

Other

Exercise and Fitness

DAILY PHYSICAL ACTIVITIES

ACTIVITY/ EXERCISE	hrs./ mins.	reps./ sets	------INTENSITY------			cal. burned
			low	med	high	
TOTAL CALORIES BURNED						

COMMENTS:

**VITAMINS &
SUPPLEMENTS**

Type:

Qty:

Type:

Qty:

Type:

Qty:

Type:

Qty:

Type:

Qty:

Type:

Qty:

Daily Assessment and Notes

OBSTACLES, SOLUTIONS AND THOUGHTS ON YOUR PROGRESS

Helpful Tips for Effective Weight-Loss

Start a moderate exercise routine by adding 10-15 minutes of aerobic activity to your daily schedule. From there, slowly increase the length of your workout to 45-60 minutes most days of the week.

Daily Nutritional Intake

FOOD AND BEVERAGES

MORNING TIME:	amt.	cal.	fat gms	protein gms	carbs. gms	fiber gms
BREAKFAST TOTALS						

COMMENTS:

AFTERNOON TIME:	amt.	cal.	fat gms	protein gms	carbs. gms	fiber gms
LUNCH TOTALS						

COMMENTS:

EVENING TIME:	amt.	cal.	fat gms	protein gms	carbs. gms	fiber gms
DINNER TOTALS						

COMMENTS:

Daily Serving Intake

_____ Fruits
# of servings

_____ Vegetables
# of servings

_____ Grains
# of servings

_____ Meat & Beans
# of servings

_____ Milk & Dairy
# of servings

_____ Oils & Sweets
# of servings

Water Intake

oz. _____

☐ low ☐ med ☐ high

ENERGY LEVELS

Daily Nutritional Intake

FOOD AND BEVERAGES

DAILY GOALS
ACHIEVED

SNACKS TIME:	amt.	cal.	fat gms	protein gms	carbs. gms	fiber gms
SNACK TOTALS						

COMMENTS:

DAILY TOTALS

Calories

Fat

Protein

Carbohydrates

Fiber

Other

Exercise and Fitness

DAILY PHYSICAL ACTIVITIES

ACTIVITY/ EXERCISE	hrs./ mins.	reps./ sets	------INTENSITY------ low	med	high	cal. burned
TOTAL CALORIES BURNED						

COMMENTS:

VITAMINS &
SUPPLEMENTS

Type:
Qty:
Type:
Qty:
Type:
Qty:
Type:
Qty:
Type:
Qty:
Type:
Qty:

Daily Assessment and Notes

OBSTACLES, SOLUTIONS AND THOUGHTS ON YOUR PROGRESS

Daily Nutritional Intake

FOOD AND BEVERAGES

**Helpful Tips
for Effective
Weight-Loss**

Instead of thinking
of dieting as
"giving up" foods,
think of it as eating
your favorite foods,
but in moderation.
Smaller portion
sizes and eating the
higher calorie foods
in small amounts
can help you lose
weight without
making you feel
like you are
depriving yourself.

MORNING TIME:	amt.	cal.	fat gms	protein gms	carbs. gms	fiber gms
BREAKFAST TOTALS						

COMMENTS:

AFTERNOON TIME:	amt.	cal.	fat gms	protein gms	carbs. gms	fiber gms
LUNCH TOTALS						

COMMENTS:

Daily Serving Intake

_____ Fruits
# of servings

_____ Vegetables
# of servings

_____ Grains
# of servings

_____ Meat & Beans
# of servings

_____ Milk & Dairy
# of servings

_____ Oils & Sweets
# of servings

EVENING TIME:	amt.	cal.	fat gms	protein gms	carbs. gms	fiber gms
DINNER TOTALS						

Water Intake

oz.

COMMENTS:

☐ low   ☐ med   ☐ high

ENERGY LEVELS

Daily Nutritional Intake

FOOD AND BEVERAGES

DAILY GOALS
ACHIEVED

SNACKS TIME:	amt.	cal.	fat gms	protein gms	carbs. gms	fiber gms
SNACK TOTALS						

COMMENTS:

DAILY TOTALS

Calories

Fat

Protein

Carbohydrates

Fiber

Other

Exercise and Fitness

DAILY PHYSICAL ACTIVITIES

ACTIVITY/ EXERCISE	hrs./ mins.	reps./ sets	------INTENSITY------ low	med	high	cal. burned
TOTAL CALORIES BURNED						

COMMENTS:

VITAMINS &
SUPPLEMENTS

Type:
Qty:
Type:
Qty:
Type:
Qty:
Type:
Qty:
Type:
Qty:
Type:
Qty:

Daily Assessment and Notes

OBSTACLES, SOLUTIONS AND THOUGHTS ON YOUR PROGRESS

WEIGHT

Daily Nutritional Intake

FOOD AND BEVERAGES

Make slow, small
changes to your
diet instead of fast,
big changes. This
way your healthy
lifestyle is easier to
maintain.

MORNING TIME:	amt.	cal.	fat gms	protein gms	carbs. gms	fiber gms
BREAKFAST TOTALS						

COMMENTS:

AFTERNOON TIME:	amt.	cal.	fat gms	protein gms	carbs. gms	fiber gms
LUNCH TOTALS						

COMMENTS:

Daily Serving Intake

____ Fruits
# of servings

____ Vegetables
# of servings

____ Grains
# of servings

____ Meat & Beans
# of servings

____ Milk & Dairy
# of servings

____ Oils & Sweets
# of servings

EVENING TIME:	amt.	cal.	fat gms	protein gms	carbs. gms	fiber gms
DINNER TOTALS						

Water Intake

oz. ____

COMMENTS:

❑ low ❑ med ❑ high

ENERGY LEVELS

Daily Nutritional Intake

FOOD AND BEVERAGES

**DAILY GOALS
ACHIEVED**

SNACKS TIME:	amt.	cal.	fat gms	protein gms	carbs. gms	fiber gms
SNACK TOTALS						

COMMENTS:

DAILY TOTALS

Calories

Fat

Protein

Carbohydrates

Fiber

Other

Exercise and Fitness

DAILY PHYSICAL ACTIVITIES

ACTIVITY/ EXERCISE	hrs./ mins.	reps./ sets	------INTENSITY------			cal. burned
			low	med	high	
TOTAL CALORIES BURNED						

COMMENTS:

**VITAMINS &
SUPPLEMENTS**

Type:

Qty:

Type:

Qty:

Type:

Qty:

Type:

Qty:

Type:

Qty:

Type:

Qty:

Daily Assessment and Notes

OBSTACLES, SOLUTIONS AND THOUGHTS ON YOUR PROGRESS

Daily Nutritional Intake

FOOD AND BEVERAGES

MORNING TIME:	amt.	cal.	fat gms	protein gms	carbs. gms	fiber gms
BREAKFAST TOTALS						

COMMENTS:

AFTERNOON TIME:	amt.	cal.	fat gms	protein gms	carbs. gms	fiber gms
LUNCH TOTALS						

COMMENTS:

EVENING TIME:	amt.	cal.	fat gms	protein gms	carbs. gms	fiber gms
DINNER TOTALS						

COMMENTS:

Daily Serving Intake

____ Fruits
# of servings

____ Vegetables
# of servings

____ Grains
# of servings

____ Meat & Beans
# of servings

____ Milk & Dairy
# of servings

____ Oils & Sweets
# of servings

Water Intake

oz.

❏ low   ❏ med   ❏ high

ENERGY LEVELS

Daily Nutritional Intake

FOOD AND BEVERAGES

DAILY GOALS
ACHIEVED

DAILY TOTALS

SNACKS TIME:	amt.	cal.	fat gms	protein gms	carbs. gms	fiber gms
SNACK TOTALS						

COMMENTS:

Calories

Fat

Protein

Carbohydrates

Fiber

Other

Exercise and Fitness

DAILY PHYSICAL ACTIVITIES

VITAMINS &
SUPPLEMENTS

ACTIVITY/ EXERCISE	hrs./ mins.	reps./ sets	------INTENSITY------ low	med	high	cal. burned
TOTAL CALORIES BURNED						

COMMENTS:

Type:
Qty:
Type:
Qty:
Type:
Qty:
Type:
Qty:
Type:
Qty:
Type:
Qty:

Daily Assessment and Notes

OBSTACLES, SOLUTIONS AND THOUGHTS ON YOUR PROGRESS

DATE   WEIGHT

**Helpful Tips
for Effective
Weight-Loss**

Working out on an
empty stomach,
such as in the
morning or before
you eat dinner, will
help you burn the
maximum amount
of fat and calories.

If you need a little
burst of energy
during your
workout, have a
snack with complex
carbohydrates and
protein handy, like
a small piece of
fruit and cheese or
whole wheat
crackers with
peanut butter.

Daily Serving Intake

_____ Fruits
       # of servings

_____ Vegetables
       # of servings

_____ Grains
       # of servings

_____ Meat & Beans
       # of servings

_____ Milk & Dairy
       # of servings

_____ Oils & Sweets
       # of servings

Water Intake

oz. _____

Daily Nutritional Intake

FOOD AND BEVERAGES

MORNING TIME:	amt.	cal.	fat gms	protein gms	carbs. gms	fiber gms
BREAKFAST TOTALS						

COMMENTS:

AFTERNOON TIME:	amt.	cal.	fat gms	protein gms	carbs. gms	fiber gms
LUNCH TOTALS						

COMMENTS:

EVENING TIME:	amt.	cal.	fat gms	protein gms	carbs. gms	fiber gms
DINNER TOTALS						

COMMENTS:

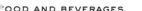

❏ low ❏ med ❏ high

ENERGY LEVELS

Daily Nutritional Intake

FOOD AND BEVERAGES

DAILY GOALS
ACHIEVED

SNACKS TIME:	amt.	cal.	fat gms	protein gms	carbs. gms	fiber gms
SNACK TOTALS						

COMMENTS:

DAILY TOTALS

Calories

Fat

Protein

Carbohydrates

Fiber

Other

Exercise and Fitness

DAILY PHYSICAL ACTIVITIES

ACTIVITY/ EXERCISE	hrs./ mins.	reps./ sets	low	med	high	cal. burned
TOTAL CALORIES BURNED						

(INTENSITY spans low, med, high)

COMMENTS:

VITAMINS &
SUPPLEMENTS

Type:
Qty:
Type:
Qty:
Type:
Qty:
Type:
Qty:
Type:
Qty:
Type:
Qty:

Daily Assessment and Notes

OBSTACLES, SOLUTIONS AND THOUGHTS ON YOUR PROGRESS

WEIGHT

Daily Nutritional Intake

FOOD AND BEVERAGES

MORNING TIME:	amt.	cal.	fat gms	protein gms	carbs. gms	fiber gms
BREAKFAST TOTALS						

COMMENTS:

AFTERNOON TIME:	amt.	cal.	fat gms	protein gms	carbs. gms	fiber gms
LUNCH TOTALS						

COMMENTS:

EVENING TIME:	amt.	cal.	fat gms	protein gms	carbs. gms	fiber gms
DINNER TOTALS						

COMMENTS:

Daily Serving Intake

____ Fruits
# of servings

____ Vegetables
# of servings

____ Grains
# of servings

____ Meat & Beans
# of servings

____ Milk & Dairy
# of servings

____ Oils & Sweets
# of servings

Water Intake

oz.

178

❏ low ❏ med ❏ high

ENERGY LEVELS

Daily Nutritional Intake

FOOD AND BEVERAGES

DAILY GOALS ACHIEVED

SNACKS TIME:	amt.	cal.	fat gms	protein gms	carbs. gms	fiber gms
SNACK TOTALS						

COMMENTS:

DAILY TOTALS

Calories

Fat

Protein

Carbohydrates

Fiber

Other

Exercise and Fitness

DAILY PHYSICAL ACTIVITIES

ACTIVITY/ EXERCISE	hrs./ mins.	reps./ sets	------INTENSITY------			cal. burned
			low	med	high	
TOTAL CALORIES BURNED						

COMMENTS:

VITAMINS & SUPPLEMENTS

Type:

Qty:

Type:

Qty:

Type:

Qty:

Type:

Qty:

Type:

Qty:

Type:

Qty:

Daily Assessment and Notes

OBSTACLES, SOLUTIONS AND THOUGHTS ON YOUR PROGRESS

WEIGHT

Helpful Tips for Effective Weight-Loss

Don't eat snack foods directly out of the package. You can easily eat much more than the standard serving size.

Measure the portion you want to eat on a plate, and put the rest away.

Daily Nutritional Intake

FOOD AND BEVERAGES

MORNING TIME:	amt.	cal.	fat gms	protein gms	carbs. gms	fiber gms
BREAKFAST TOTALS						

COMMENTS:

AFTERNOON TIME:	amt.	cal.	fat gms	protein gms	carbs. gms	fiber gms
LUNCH TOTALS						

COMMENTS:

Daily Serving Intake

____ Fruits
# of servings

____ Vegetables
# of servings

____ Grains
# of servings

____ Meat & Beans
# of servings

____ Milk & Dairy
# of servings

____ Oils & Sweets
# of servings

Water Intake

oz. _____

EVENING TIME:	amt.	cal.	fat gms	protein gms	carbs. gms	fiber gms
DINNER TOTALS						

COMMENTS:

180

❏ low ❏ med ❏ high

ENERGY LEVELS

Daily Nutritional Intake

FOOD AND BEVERAGES

DAILY GOALS
ACHIEVED

SNACKS TIME:	amt.	cal.	fat gms	protein gms	carbs. gms	fiber gms
SNACK TOTALS						

COMMENTS:

DAILY TOTALS

Calories

Fat

Protein

Carbohydrates

Fiber

Other

Exercise and Fitness

DAILY PHYSICAL ACTIVITIES

ACTIVITY/ EXERCISE	hrs./ mins.	reps./ sets	------INTENSITY------			cal. burned
			low	med	high	
TOTAL CALORIES BURNED						

COMMENTS:

VITAMINS &
SUPPLEMENTS

Type:
Qty:
Type:
Qty:
Type:
Qty:
Type:
Qty:
Type:
Qty:
Type:
Qty:

Daily Assessment and Notes

OBSTACLES, SOLUTIONS AND THOUGHTS ON YOUR PROGRESS

Helpful Tips
for Effective
Weight-Loss

It takes 20 minutes
for your brain to
register that your
stomach is full. If
you eat slower
while enjoying
every bite, you
are less likely to
overeat.

Daily Nutritional Intake

FOOD AND BEVERAGES

MORNING TIME:	amt.	cal.	fat gms	protein gms	carbs. gms	fiber gms
BREAKFAST TOTALS						

COMMENTS:

AFTERNOON TIME:	amt.	cal.	fat gms	protein gms	carbs. gms	fiber gms
LUNCH TOTALS						

COMMENTS:

Daily Serving Intake

_____ Fruits
# of servings

_____ Vegetables
# of servings

_____ Grains
# of servings

_____ Meat & Beans
# of servings

_____ Milk & Dairy
# of servings

_____ Oils & Sweets
# of servings

Water Intake

oz.

EVENING TIME:	amt.	cal.	fat gms	protein gms	carbs. gms	fiber gms
DINNER TOTALS						

COMMENTS:

Daily Nutritional Intake

FOOD AND BEVERAGES

DAILY GOALS
ACHIEVED

SNACKS TIME:	amt.	cal.	fat gms	protein gms	carbs. gms	fiber gms
SNACK TOTALS						

COMMENTS:

DAILY TOTALS

Calories

Fat

Protein

Carbohydrates

Fiber

Other

Exercise and Fitness

DAILY PHYSICAL ACTIVITIES

ACTIVITY/ EXERCISE	hrs./ mins.	reps./ sets	------INTENSITY------ low	med	high	cal. burned
TOTAL CALORIES BURNED						

COMMENTS:

VITAMINS &
SUPPLEMENTS

Type:
Qty:

Type:
Qty:

Type:
Qty:

Type:
Qty:

Type:
Qty:

Type:
Qty:

Daily Assessment and Notes

OBSTACLES, SOLUTIONS AND THOUGHTS ON YOUR PROGRESS

DATE

Daily Nutritional Intake

FOOD AND BEVERAGES

MORNING TIME:	amt.	cal.	fat gms	protein gms	carbs. gms	fiber gms
BREAKFAST TOTALS						

COMMENTS:

AFTERNOON TIME:	amt.	cal.	fat gms	protein gms	carbs. gms	fiber gms
LUNCH TOTALS						

COMMENTS:

Daily Serving Intake

____ Fruits
 # of servings

____ Vegetables
 # of servings

____ Grains
 # of servings

____ Meat & Beans
 # of servings

____ Milk & Dairy
 # of servings

____ Oils & Sweets
 # of servings

Water Intake

oz.

EVENING TIME:	amt.	cal.	fat gms	protein gms	carbs. gms	fiber gms
DINNER TOTALS						

COMMENTS:

184

❏ low   ❏ med   ❏ high

ENERGY LEVELS

Daily Nutritional Intake

FOOD AND BEVERAGES

DAILY GOALS
ACHIEVED

DAILY TOTALS

SNACKS TIME:	amt.	cal.	fat gms	protein gms	carbs. gms	fiber gms
SNACK TOTALS						

COMMENTS:

Calories

Fat

Protein

Carbohydrates

Fiber

Other

Exercise and Fitness

DAILY PHYSICAL ACTIVITIES

VITAMINS &
SUPPLEMENTS

ACTIVITY/ EXERCISE	hrs./ mins.	reps./ sets	------INTENSITY------			cal. burned
			low	med	high	
TOTAL CALORIES BURNED						

COMMENTS:

Type:
Qty:
Type:
Qty:
Type:
Qty:
Type:
Qty:
Type:
Qty:
Type:
Qty:

Daily Assessment and Notes

OBSTACLES, SOLUTIONS AND THOUGHTS ON YOUR PROGRESS

Helpful Tips
for Effective
Weight-Loss

Tofu is a good
substitute for many
foods because it is
rich in high-quality
protein, a good
source of B-vita-
mins and iron, and
contains no choles-
terol.

Try using it in place
of cream in sauces
or as a substitute
for soft cheeses in
recipes such as
lasagna.

Daily Nutritional Intake

FOOD AND BEVERAGES

MORNING TIME:		amt.	cal.	fat gms	protein gms	carbs. gms	fiber gms
BREAKFAST TOTALS							

COMMENTS:

AFTERNOON TIME:		amt.	cal.	fat gms	protein gms	carbs. gms	fiber gms
LUNCH TOTALS							

COMMENTS:

Daily Serving Intake

_____ Fruits
  # of servings

_____ Vegetables
  # of servings

_____ Grains
  # of servings

_____ Meat & Beans
  # of servings

_____ Milk & Dairy
  # of servings

_____ Oils & Sweets
  # of servings

EVENING TIME:		amt.	cal.	fat gms	protein gms	carbs. gms	fiber gms
DINNER TOTALS							

COMMENTS:

Water Intake

oz.

Daily Nutritional Intake

FOOD AND BEVERAGES

**DAILY GOALS
ACHIEVED**

SNACKS TIME:	amt.	cal.	fat gms	protein gms	carbs. gms	fiber gms
SNACK TOTALS						

COMMENTS:

DAILY TOTALS

Calories

Fat

Protein

Carbohydrates

Fiber

Other

Exercise and Fitness

DAILY PHYSICAL ACTIVITIES

ACTIVITY/ EXERCISE	hrs./ mins.	reps./ sets	------INTENSITY------			cal. burned
			low	med	high	
TOTAL CALORIES BURNED						

COMMENTS:

**VITAMINS &
SUPPLEMENTS**

Type:

Qty:

Type:

Qty:

Type:

Qty:

Type:

Qty:

Type:

Qty:

Type:

Qty:

Daily Assessment and Notes

OBSTACLES, SOLUTIONS AND THOUGHTS ON YOUR PROGRESS

WEIGHT

Helpful Tips
for Effective
Weight-Loss

Daily Nutritional Intake

FOOD AND BEVERAGES

Chicken broth and
fresh herbs are an
excellent and
delicious substitute
for butter and
margarine when
cooking.

MORNING TIME:	amt.	cal.	fat gms	protein gms	carbs. gms	fiber gms
BREAKFAST TOTALS						

COMMENTS:

AFTERNOON TIME:	amt.	cal.	fat gms	protein gms	carbs. gms	fiber gms
LUNCH TOTALS						

COMMENTS:

Daily Serving Intake

_____ Fruits
# of servings

_____ Vegetables
# of servings

_____ Grains
# of servings

_____ Meat & Beans
# of servings

_____ Milk & Dairy
# of servings

_____ Oils & Sweets
# of servings

Water Intake

oz.

EVENING TIME:	amt.	cal.	fat gms	protein gms	carbs. gms	fiber gms
DINNER TOTALS						

COMMENTS:

❏ low ❏ med ❏ high

ENERGY LEVELS

Daily Nutritional Intake

FOOD AND BEVERAGES

**DAILY GOALS
ACHIEVED**

SNACKS TIME:	amt.	cal.	fat gms	protein gms	carbs. gms	fiber gms
SNACK TOTALS						

COMMENTS:

DAILY TOTALS

Calories

Fat

Protein

Carbohydrates

Fiber

Other

Exercise and Fitness

DAILY PHYSICAL ACTIVITIES

ACTIVITY/ EXERCISE	hrs./ mins.	reps./ sets	------INTENSITY------ low	med	high	cal. burned
TOTAL CALORIES BURNED						

COMMENTS:

**VITAMINS &
SUPPLEMENTS**

Type:
Qty:
Type:
Qty:
Type:
Qty:
Type:
Qty:
Type:
Qty:
Type:
Qty:

Daily Assessment and Notes

OBSTACLES, SOLUTIONS AND THOUGHTS ON YOUR PROGRESS

189

WEIGHT

Daily Nutritional Intake

FOOD AND BEVERAGES

After dinner or
other large meals,
try going for a long
walk with a friend
if the weather is
permitting.

MORNING TIME:	amt.	cal.	fat gms	protein gms	carbs. gms	fiber gms
BREAKFAST TOTALS						

COMMENTS:

AFTERNOON TIME:	amt.	cal.	fat gms	protein gms	carbs. gms	fiber gms
LUNCH TOTALS						

COMMENTS:

Daily Serving Intake

_____ Fruits
# of servings

_____ Vegetables
# of servings

_____ Grains
# of servings

EVENING TIME:	amt.	cal.	fat gms	protein gms	carbs. gms	fiber gms
DINNER TOTALS						

_____ Meat & Beans
# of servings

_____ Milk & Dairy
# of servings

_____ Oils & Sweets
# of servings

Water Intake

oz. _____

COMMENTS:

❏ low ❏ med ❏ high

ENERGY LEVELS

Daily Nutritional Intake

FOOD AND BEVERAGES

DAILY TOTALS

SNACKS TIME:	amt.	cal.	fat gms	protein gms	carbs. gms	fiber gms
SNACK TOTALS						

COMMENTS:

Calories

Fat

Protein

Carbohydrates

Fiber

Other

Exercise and Fitness

DAILY PHYSICAL ACTIVITIES

VITAMINS &
SUPPLEMENTS

ACTIVITY/ EXERCISE	hrs./ mins.	reps./ sets	------INTENSITY------			cal. burned
			low	med	high	
TOTAL CALORIES BURNED						

COMMENTS:

Type:

Qty:

Type:

Qty:

Type:

Qty:

Type:

Qty:

Type:

Qty:

Type:

Qty:

Daily Assessment and Notes

OBSTACLES, SOLUTIONS AND THOUGHTS ON YOUR PROGRESS

DATE

WEIGHT

Helpful Tips
for Effective
Weight-Loss

Each time you sit
down to eat, think
of it as a new
opportunity to
make healthy food
choices!

Daily Nutritional Intake

FOOD AND BEVERAGES

MORNING TIME:	amt.	cal.	fat gms	protein gms	carbs. gms	fiber gms
BREAKFAST TOTALS						

COMMENTS:

AFTERNOON TIME:	amt.	cal.	fat gms	protein gms	carbs. gms	fiber gms
LUNCH TOTALS						

COMMENTS:

EVENING TIME:	amt.	cal.	fat gms	protein gms	carbs. gms	fiber gms
DINNER TOTALS						

COMMENTS:

Daily Serving Intake

____ Fruits
# of servings

____ Vegetables
# of servings

____ Grains
# of servings

____ Meat & Beans
# of servings

____ Milk & Dairy
# of servings

____ Oils & Sweets
# of servings

Water Intake

oz.

192

❏ low　❏ med　❏ high

ENERGY LEVELS

Daily Nutritional Intake

FOOD AND BEVERAGES

SNACKS TIME:	amt.	cal.	fat gms	protein gms	carbs. gms	fiber gms
SNACK TOTALS						

COMMENTS:

DAILY TOTALS

Calories

Fat

Protein

Carbohydrates

Fiber

Other

Exercise and Fitness

DAILY PHYSICAL ACTIVITIES

ACTIVITY/ EXERCISE	hrs./ mins.	reps./ sets	------INTENSITY------			cal. burned
			low	med	high	
TOTAL CALORIES BURNED						

COMMENTS:

VITAMINS & SUPPLEMENTS

Type:

Qty:

Type:

Qty:

Type:

Qty:

Type:

Qty:

Type:

Qty:

Type:

Qty:

Daily Assessment and Notes

OBSTACLES, SOLUTIONS AND THOUGHTS ON YOUR PROGRESS

WEIGHT

Daily Nutritional Intake

FOOD AND BEVERAGES

Try to choose
snacks that are rich
in vitamins and will
give you the proper
nutrients your body
needs. That way,
you won't just be
consuming empty
calories.

MORNING TIME:	amt.	cal.	fat gms	protein gms	carbs. gms	fiber gms
BREAKFAST TOTALS						

COMMENTS:

AFTERNOON TIME:	amt.	cal.	fat gms	protein gms	carbs. gms	fiber gms
LUNCH TOTALS						

COMMENTS:

Daily Serving Intake

____ Fruits
# of servings

____ Vegetables
# of servings

____ Grains
# of servings

____ Meat & Beans
# of servings

____ Milk & Dairy
# of servings

____ Oils & Sweets
# of servings

Water Intake

oz.

EVENING TIME:	amt.	cal.	fat gms	protein gms	carbs. gms	fiber gms
DINNER TOTALS						

COMMENTS:

☐ low ☐ med ☐ high

ENERGY LEVELS

Daily Nutritional Intake

FOOD AND BEVERAGES

DAILY GOALS
ACHIEVED

DAILY TOTALS

SNACKS TIME:	amt.	cal.	fat gms	protein gms	carbs. gms	fiber gms
SNACK TOTALS						

COMMENTS:

Calories

Fat

Protein

Carbohydrates

Fiber

Other

Exercise and Fitness

DAILY PHYSICAL ACTIVITIES

VITAMINS &
SUPPLEMENTS

ACTIVITY/ EXERCISE	hrs./ mins.	reps./ sets	------INTENSITY------			cal. burned
			low	med	high	
TOTAL CALORIES BURNED						

COMMENTS:

Type:
Qty:
Type:
Qty:
Type:
Qty:
Type:
Qty:
Type:
Qty:
Type:
Qty:

Daily Assessment and Notes

OBSTACLES, SOLUTIONS AND THOUGHTS ON YOUR PROGRESS

WEIGHT

Helpful Tips
for Effective
Weight-Loss

Daily Nutritional Intake

FOOD AND BEVERAGES

Buy a healthy
cookbook or food
magazine. It will
be filled with
delicious recipes to
help you cook
healthier meals.

MORNING TIME:	amt.	cal.	fat gms	protein gms	carbs. gms	fiber gms
BREAKFAST TOTALS						

COMMENTS:

AFTERNOON TIME:	amt.	cal.	fat gms	protein gms	carbs. gms	fiber gms
LUNCH TOTALS						

COMMENTS:

Daily Serving Intake

____ Fruits
# of servings

____ Vegetables
# of servings

____ Grains
# of servings

____ Meat & Beans
# of servings

____ Milk & Dairy
# of servings

____ Oils & Sweets
# of servings

EVENING TIME:	amt.	cal.	fat gms	protein gms	carbs. gms	fiber gms
DINNER TOTALS						

Water Intake

COMMENTS:

oz. _____

☐ low ☐ med ☐ high

ENERGY LEVELS

DAILY GOALS
ACHIEVED

Daily Nutritional Intake

FOOD AND BEVERAGES

DAILY TOTALS

SNACKS TIME:	amt.	cal.	fat gms	protein gms	carbs. gms	fiber gms
SNACK TOTALS						

COMMENTS:

Calories

Fat

Protein

Carbohydrates

Fiber

Other

Exercise and Fitness

DAILY PHYSICAL ACTIVITIES

ACTIVITY/ EXERCISE	hrs./ mins.	reps./ sets	------INTENSITY------ low	med	high	cal. burned
TOTAL CALORIES BURNED						

COMMENTS:

VITAMINS &
SUPPLEMENTS

Type:

Qty:

Type:

Qty:

Type:

Qty:

Type:

Qty:

Type:

Qty:

Type:

Qty:

Daily Assessment and Notes

OBSTACLES, SOLUTIONS AND THOUGHTS ON YOUR PROGRESS

Helpful Tips
for Effective
Weight-Loss

When possible,
take the stairs or
park further away
from the store.
Extra steps in your
day mean extra
calories burned
over the long run.

Daily Nutritional Intake

FOOD AND BEVERAGES

MORNING TIME:	amt.	cal.	fat gms	protein gms	carbs. gms	fiber gms
BREAKFAST TOTALS						

COMMENTS:

AFTERNOON TIME:	amt.	cal.	fat gms	protein gms	carbs. gms	fiber gms
LUNCH TOTALS						

COMMENTS:

Daily Serving Intake

_____ Fruits
# of servings

_____ Vegetables
# of servings

_____ Grains
# of servings

_____ Meat & Beans
# of servings

_____ Milk & Dairy
# of servings

_____ Oils & Sweets
# of servings

Water Intake

oz.

EVENING TIME:	amt.	cal.	fat gms	protein gms	carbs. gms	fiber gms
DINNER TOTALS						

COMMENTS:

☐ low ☐ med ☐ high

ENERGY LEVELS

Daily Nutritional Intake

FOOD AND BEVERAGES

**DAILY GOALS
ACHIEVED**

DAILY TOTALS

SNACKS TIME:		amt.	cal.	fat gms	protein gms	carbs. gms	fiber gms
SNACK TOTALS							

COMMENTS:

Calories

Fat

Protein

Carbohydrates

Fiber

Other

Exercise and Fitness

DAILY PHYSICAL ACTIVITIES

**VITAMINS &
SUPPLEMENTS**

ACTIVITY/ EXERCISE		hrs./ mins.	reps./ sets	------INTENSITY------ low	med	high	cal. burned
TOTAL CALORIES BURNED							

COMMENTS:

Type:

Qty:

Type:

Qty:

Type:

Qty:

Type:

Qty:

Type:

Qty:

Type:

Qty:

Daily Assessment and Notes

OBSTACLES, SOLUTIONS AND THOUGHTS ON YOUR PROGRESS

DATE

Daily Nutritional Intake

**Helpful Tips
for Effective
Weight-Loss**

If joining a gym is
not your thing, try
organizing a pickup
game of basketball
or Frisbee. Take a
jog outdoors or
walk your dog, if
the weather is nice.

MORNING TIME:	amt.	cal.	fat gms	protein gms	carbs. gms	fiber gms
BREAKFAST TOTALS						

COMMENTS:

AFTERNOON TIME:	amt.	cal.	fat gms	protein gms	carbs. gms	fiber gms
LUNCH TOTALS						

COMMENTS:

Daily Serving Intake

_____ Fruits
\# of servings

_____ Vegetables
\# of servings

_____ Grains
\# of servings

_____ Meat & Beans
\# of servings

_____ Milk & Dairy
\# of servings

_____ Oils & Sweets
\# of servings

Water Intake

\# oz.

EVENING TIME:	amt.	cal.	fat gms	protein gms	carbs. gms	fiber gms
DINNER TOTALS						

COMMENTS:

200

☐ low   ☐ med   ☐ high

ENERGY LEVELS

Daily Nutritional Intake

FOOD AND BEVERAGES

**DAILY GOALS
ACHIEVED**

SNACKS TIME:	amt.	cal.	fat gms	protein gms	carbs. gms	fiber gms
SNACK TOTALS						

COMMENTS:

DAILY TOTALS

Calories

Fat

Protein

Carbohydrates

Fiber

Other

Exercise and Fitness

DAILY PHYSICAL ACTIVITIES

ACTIVITY/ EXERCISE	hrs./ mins.	reps./ sets	------INTENSITY------			cal. burned
			low	med	high	
TOTAL CALORIES BURNED						

COMMENTS:

**VITAMINS &
SUPPLEMENTS**

Type:

Qty:

Type:

Qty:

Type:

Qty:

Type:

Qty:

Type:

Qty:

Type:

Qty:

Daily Assessment and Notes

OBSTACLES, SOLUTIONS AND THOUGHTS ON YOUR PROGRESS

WEIGHT

Helpful Tips
for Effective
Weight-Loss

Daily Nutritional Intake

FOOD AND BEVERAGES

Focus on the
positive: don't
think of how much
more weight you
have to lose, think
about how much
you've already lost!
Congratulate your-
self every time you
get a step closer to
your goal.

MORNING TIME:	amt.	cal.	fat gms	protein gms	carbs. gms	fiber gms
BREAKFAST TOTALS						

COMMENTS:

AFTERNOON TIME:	amt.	cal.	fat gms	protein gms	carbs. gms	fiber gms
LUNCH TOTALS						

COMMENTS:

Daily Serving Intake

_____ Fruits
# of servings

_____ Vegetables
# of servings

_____ Grains
# of servings

EVENING TIME:	amt.	cal.	fat gms	protein gms	carbs. gms	fiber gms
DINNER TOTALS						

_____ Meat & Beans
# of servings

_____ Milk & Dairy
# of servings

_____ Oils & Sweets
# of servings

Water Intake

oz.

COMMENTS:

☐ low   ☐ med   ☐ high

ENERGY LEVELS

Daily Nutritional Intake

FOOD AND BEVERAGES

**DAILY GOALS
ACHIEVED**

DAILY TOTALS

SNACKS TIME:		amt.	cal.	fat gms	protein gms	carbs. gms	fiber gms
SNACK TOTALS							

COMMENTS:

Calories

Fat

Protein

Carbohydrates

Fiber

Other

Exercise and Fitness

DAILY PHYSICAL ACTIVITIES

VITAMINS &

SUPPLEMENTS

ACTIVITY/ EXERCISE		hrs./ mins.	reps./ sets	------INTENSITY------			cal. burned
				low	med	high	
TOTAL CALORIES BURNED							

COMMENTS:

Type:

Qty:

Type:

Qty:

Type:

Qty:

Type:

Qty:

Type:

Qty:

Type:

Qty:

Daily Assessment and Notes

OBSTACLES, SOLUTIONS AND THOUGHTS ON YOUR PROGRESS

_____

_____

_____

_____

_____

Daily Nutritional Intake

FOOD AND BEVERAGES

MORNING TIME:	amt.	cal.	fat gms	protein gms	carbs. gms	fiber gms
BREAKFAST TOTALS						

COMMENTS:

AFTERNOON TIME:	amt.	cal.	fat gms	protein gms	carbs. gms	fiber gms
LUNCH TOTALS						

COMMENTS:

Daily Serving Intake

_____ Fruits
# of servings

_____ Vegetables
# of servings

_____ Grains
# of servings

_____ Meat & Beans
# of servings

_____ Milk & Dairy
# of servings

_____ Oils & Sweets
# of servings

EVENING TIME:	amt.	cal.	fat gms	protein gms	carbs. gms	fiber gms
DINNER TOTALS						

COMMENTS:

Water Intake

oz.

Daily Nutritional Intake

FOOD AND BEVERAGES

**DAILY GOALS
ACHIEVED**

DAILY TOTALS

SNACKS TIME:	amt.	cal.	fat gms	protein gms	carbs. gms	fiber gms
SNACK TOTALS						

COMMENTS:

Calories

Fat

Protein

Carbohydrates

Fiber

Other

Exercise and Fitness

DAILY PHYSICAL ACTIVITIES

**VITAMINS &
SUPPLEMENTS**

ACTIVITY/ EXERCISE	hrs./ mins.	reps./ sets	------INTENSITY------			cal. burned
			low	med	high	
TOTAL CALORIES BURNED						

COMMENTS:

Type:

Qty:

Type:

Qty:

Type:

Qty:

Type:

Qty:

Type:

Qty:

Type:

Qty:

Daily Assessment and Notes

OBSTACLES, SOLUTIONS AND THOUGHTS ON YOUR PROGRESS

DATE

Daily Nutritional Intake

**Helpful Tips
for Effective
Weight-Loss**

Avoid going to a
candy store or an
ice cream shop,
where you will be
tempted to stray
from your diet.

FOOD AND BEVERAGES

MORNING TIME:	amt.	cal.	fat gms	protein gms	carbs. gms	fiber gms
BREAKFAST TOTALS						

COMMENTS:

AFTERNOON TIME:	amt.	cal.	fat gms	protein gms	carbs. gms	fiber gms
LUNCH TOTALS						

COMMENTS:

Daily Serving Intake

_____ Fruits
# of servings

_____ Vegetables
# of servings

_____ Grains
# of servings

_____ Meat & Beans
# of servings

_____ Milk & Dairy
# of servings

_____ Oils & Sweets
# of servings

EVENING TIME:	amt.	cal.	fat gms	protein gms	carbs. gms	fiber gms
DINNER TOTALS						

Water Intake

oz.

COMMENTS:

ENERGY LEVELS

Daily Nutritional Intake

FOOD AND BEVERAGES

DAILY GOALS ACHIEVED

DAILY TOTALS

SNACKS TIME:	amt.	cal.	fat gms	protein gms	carbs. gms	fiber gms
SNACK TOTALS						

COMMENTS:

Calories

Fat

Protein

Carbohydrates

Fiber

Other

Exercise and Fitness

DAILY PHYSICAL ACTIVITIES

VITAMINS & SUPPLEMENTS

ACTIVITY/ EXERCISE	hrs./ mins.	reps./ sets	low	med	high	cal. burned
TOTAL CALORIES BURNED						

------INTENSITY------

COMMENTS:

Type:
Qty:
Type:
Qty:
Type:
Qty:
Type:
Qty:
Type:
Qty:
Type:
Qty:

Daily Assessment and Notes

OBSTACLES, SOLUTIONS AND THOUGHTS ON YOUR PROGRESS

Daily Nutritional Intake

Helpful Tips
for Effective
Weight-Loss

FOOD AND BEVERAGES

MORNING TIME:		amt.	cal.	fat gms	protein gms	carbs. gms	fiber gms
BREAKFAST TOTALS							

COMMENTS:

If you don't like
running, try
walking!

Walking at least 3
miles a day can
contribute signifi-
cantly to your
weight-loss
program.

AFTERNOON TIME:		amt.	cal.	fat gms	protein gms	carbs. gms	fiber gms
LUNCH TOTALS							

COMMENTS:

Daily Serving Intake

_____ Fruits
     # of servings

_____ Vegetables
     # of servings

_____ Grains
     # of servings

EVENING TIME:		amt.	cal.	fat gms	protein gms	carbs. gms	fiber gms
DINNER TOTALS							

COMMENTS:

_____ Meat & Beans
     # of servings

_____ Milk & Dairy
     # of servings

_____ Oils & Sweets
     # of servings

Water Intake

oz. _____

Daily Nutritional Intake

FOOD AND BEVERAGES

DAILY GOALS ACHIEVED

SNACKS TIME:	amt.	cal.	fat gms	protein gms	carbs. gms	fiber gms
SNACK TOTALS						

COMMENTS:

DAILY TOTALS

Calories

Fat

Protein

Carbohydrates

Fiber

Other

Exercise and Fitness

DAILY PHYSICAL ACTIVITIES

ACTIVITY/ EXERCISE	hrs./ mins.	reps./ sets	------INTENSITY------ low	med	high	cal. burned
TOTAL CALORIES BURNED						

COMMENTS:

VITAMINS & SUPPLEMENTS

Type:
Qty:
Type:
Qty:
Type:
Qty:
Type:
Qty:
Type:
Qty:
Type:
Qty:
Type:
Qty:

Daily Assessment and Notes

OBSTACLES, SOLUTIONS AND THOUGHTS ON YOUR PROGRESS

WEIGHT

Helpful Tips
for Effective
Weight-Loss

Daily Nutritional Intake

FOOD AND BEVERAGES

Add strength
training to your
aerobic workout.
You will burn fat
faster in the areas
you build muscle.

MORNING TIME:		amt.	cal.	fat gms	protein gms	carbs. gms	fiber gms
BREAKFAST TOTALS							

COMMENTS:

AFTERNOON TIME:		amt.	cal.	fat gms	protein gms	carbs. gms	fiber gms
LUNCH TOTALS							

COMMENTS:

Daily Serving Intake

_____ Fruits
# of servings

_____ Vegetables
# of servings

_____ Grains
# of servings

_____ Meat & Beans
# of servings

_____ Milk & Dairy
# of servings

_____ Oils & Sweets
# of servings

EVENING TIME:		amt.	cal.	fat gms	protein gms	carbs. gms	fiber gms
DINNER TOTALS							

COMMENTS:

Water Intake

oz.

■ low ☐ med ☐ high

Daily Nutritional Intake

FOOD AND BEVERAGES

DAILY GOALS
ACHIEVED

SNACKS TIME:	amt.	cal.	fat gms	protein gms	carbs. gms	fiber gms
SNACK TOTALS						

COMMENTS:

DAILY TOTALS

Calories

Fat

Protein

Carbohydrates

Fiber

Other

Exercise and Fitness

DAILY PHYSICAL ACTIVITIES

ACTIVITY/ EXERCISE	hrs./ mins.	reps./ sets	low	med	high	cal. burned
TOTAL CALORIES BURNED						

Column group header: ------INTENSITY------ (low, med, high)

COMMENTS:

VITAMINS & SUPPLEMENTS

Type:

Qty:

Type:

Qty:

Type:

Qty:

Type:

Qty:

Type:

Qty:

Type:

Qty:

Daily Assessment and Notes

OBSTACLES, SOLUTIONS AND THOUGHTS ON YOUR PROGRESS

WEIGHT

Daily Nutritional Intake

FOOD AND BEVERAGES

Before beginning
strength training at
your gym, consult a
trainer who can
guide you in the
safety procedures
and correct way to
use the machines.

MORNING TIME:	amt.	cal.	fat gms	protein gms	carbs. gms	fiber gms
BREAKFAST TOTALS						

COMMENTS:

AFTERNOON TIME:	amt.	cal.	fat gms	protein gms	carbs. gms	fiber gms
LUNCH TOTALS						

COMMENTS:

Daily Serving Intake

_____ Fruits
       # of servings

_____ Vegetables
       # of servings

_____ Grains
       # of servings

EVENING TIME:	amt.	cal.	fat gms	protein gms	carbs. gms	fiber gms
DINNER TOTALS						

_____ Meat & Beans
       # of servings

_____ Milk & Dairy
       # of servings

_____ Oils & Sweets
       # of servings

Water Intake

oz.

COMMENTS:

**DAILY GOALS
ACHIEVED**

Daily Nutritional Intake

FOOD AND BEVERAGES

DAILY TOTALS

SNACKS TIME:	amt.	cal.	fat gms	protein gms	carbs. gms	fiber gms
SNACK TOTALS						

COMMENTS:

Calories

Fat

Protein

Carbohydrates

Fiber

Other

Exercise and Fitness

DAILY PHYSICAL ACTIVITIES

ACTIVITY/ EXERCISE	hrs./ mins.	reps./ sets	------INTENSITY------ low	med	high	cal. burned
TOTAL CALORIES BURNED						

COMMENTS:

**VITAMINS &
SUPPLEMENTS**

Type:

Qty:

Type:

Qty:

Type:

Qty:

Type:

Qty:

Type:

Qty:

Type:

Qty:

Daily Assessment and Notes

OBSTACLES, SOLUTIONS AND THOUGHTS ON YOUR PROGRESS

**Helpful Tips
for Effective
Weight-Loss**

Don't cut too
many calories out
of your diet. If you
feel deprived or
unsatisfied, you are
more likely to
cheat. Keep your
calorie-limit at a
safe number.

Daily Nutritional Intake

FOOD AND BEVERAGES

MORNING TIME:	amt.	cal.	fat gms	protein gms	carbs. gms	fiber gms
BREAKFAST TOTALS						

COMMENTS:

AFTERNOON TIME:	amt.	cal.	fat gms	protein gms	carbs. gms	fiber gms
LUNCH TOTALS						

COMMENTS:

Daily Serving Intake

_____ Fruits
# of servings

_____ Vegetables
# of servings

_____ Grains
# of servings

_____ Meat & Beans
# of servings

_____ Milk & Dairy
# of servings

_____ Oils & Sweets
# of servings

EVENING TIME:	amt.	cal.	fat gms	protein gms	carbs. gms	fiber gms
DINNER TOTALS						

COMMENTS:

Water Intake

oz.

☐ low ☐ med ☐ high

ENERGY LEVELS

Daily Nutritional Intake

FOOD AND BEVERAGES

DAILY GOALS
ACHIEVED

SNACKS TIME:	amt.	cal.	fat gms	protein gms	carbs. gms	fiber gms
SNACK TOTALS						

COMMENTS:

DAILY TOTALS

Calories

Fat

Protein

Carbohydrates

Fiber

Other

Exercise and Fitness

DAILY PHYSICAL ACTIVITIES

VITAMINS &
SUPPLEMENTS

ACTIVITY/ EXERCISE	hrs./ mins.	reps./ sets	------INTENSITY------			cal. burned
			low	med	high	
TOTAL CALORIES BURNED						

COMMENTS:

Type:

Qty:

Type:

Qty:

Type:

Qty:

Type:

Qty:

Type:

Qty:

Type:

Qty:

Daily Assessment and Notes

OBSTACLES, SOLUTIONS AND THOUGHTS ON YOUR PROGRESS

WEIGHT

Daily Nutritional Intake

FOOD AND BEVERAGES

MORNING TIME:	amt.	cal.	fat gms	protein gms	carbs. gms	fiber gms
BREAKFAST TOTALS						

COMMENTS:

AFTERNOON TIME:	amt.	cal.	fat gms	protein gms	carbs. gms	fiber gms
LUNCH TOTALS						

COMMENTS:

Daily Serving Intake

____ Fruits
# of servings

____ Vegetables
# of servings

____ Grains
# of servings

____ Meat & Beans
# of servings

____ Milk & Dairy
# of servings

____ Oils & Sweets
# of servings

Water Intake

oz.

EVENING TIME:	amt.	cal.	fat gms	protein gms	carbs. gms	fiber gms
DINNER TOTALS						

COMMENTS:

☐ low ☐ med ☐ high

ENERGY LEVELS

Daily Nutritional Intake

FOOD AND BEVERAGES

**DAILY GOALS
ACHIEVED**

DAILY TOTALS

SNACKS TIME:	amt.	cal.	fat gms	protein gms	carbs. gms	fiber gms
SNACK TOTALS						

COMMENTS:

Calories

Fat

Protein

Carbohydrates

Fiber

Other

Exercise and Fitness

DAILY PHYSICAL ACTIVITIES

**VITAMINS &
SUPPLEMENTS**

ACTIVITY/ EXERCISE	hrs./ mins.	reps./ sets	------INTENSITY------ low	med	high	cal. burned
TOTAL CALORIES BURNED						

COMMENTS:

Type:
Qty:
Type:
Qty:
Type:
Qty:
Type:
Qty:
Type:
Qty:
Type:
Qty:

Daily Assessment and Notes

OBSTACLES, SOLUTIONS AND THOUGHTS ON YOUR PROGRESS

Daily Nutritional Intake

Helpful Tips for Effective Weight-Loss

Look into joining fitness classes at your local gym. Working out with other people is a great way to stay motivated.

FOOD AND BEVERAGES

MORNING TIME:	amt.	cal.	fat gms	protein gms	carbs. gms	fiber gms
BREAKFAST TOTALS						

COMMENTS:

AFTERNOON TIME:	amt.	cal.	fat gms	protein gms	carbs. gms	fiber gms
LUNCH TOTALS						

COMMENTS:

Daily Serving Intake

_____ Fruits
# of servings

_____ Vegetables
# of servings

_____ Grains
# of servings

_____ Meat & Beans
# of servings

_____ Milk & Dairy
# of servings

_____ Oils & Sweets
# of servings

Water Intake

oz.

EVENING TIME:	amt.	cal.	fat gms	protein gms	carbs. gms	fiber gms
DINNER TOTALS						

COMMENTS:

DAILY GOALS ACHIEVED

Daily Nutritional Intake

FOOD AND BEVERAGES

SNACKS TIME:	amt.	cal.	fat gms	protein gms	carbs. gms	fiber gms
SNACK TOTALS						

COMMENTS:

DAILY TOTALS

Calories

Fat

Protein

Carbohydrates

Fiber

Other

Exercise and Fitness

DAILY PHYSICAL ACTIVITIES

ACTIVITY/ EXERCISE	hrs./ mins.	reps./ sets	low	med	high	cal. burned
TOTAL CALORIES BURNED						

------INTENSITY------

COMMENTS:

VITAMINS &
SUPPLEMENTS

Type:
Qty:
Type:
Qty:
Type:
Qty:
Type:
Qty:
Type:
Qty:
Type:
Qty:

Daily Assessment and Notes

OBSTACLES, SOLUTIONS AND THOUGHTS ON YOUR PROGRESS

Daily Nutritional Intake

FOOD AND BEVERAGES

MORNING TIME:	amt.	cal.	fat gms	protein gms	carbs. gms	fiber gms
BREAKFAST TOTALS						

COMMENTS:

AFTERNOON TIME:	amt.	cal.	fat gms	protein gms	carbs. gms	fiber gms
LUNCH TOTALS						

COMMENTS:

Daily Serving Intake

____ Fruits
# of servings

____ Vegetables
# of servings

____ Grains
# of servings

____ Meat & Beans
# of servings

____ Milk & Dairy
# of servings

____ Oils & Sweets
# of servings

Water Intake

oz.

EVENING TIME:	amt.	cal.	fat gms	protein gms	carbs. gms	fiber gms
DINNER TOTALS						

COMMENTS:

☐ low ☐ med ☐ high

ENERGY LEVELS

Daily Nutritional Intake

FOOD AND BEVERAGES

DAILY GOALS
ACHIEVED

SNACKS TIME:	amt.	cal.	fat gms	protein gms	carbs. gms	fiber gms
SNACK TOTALS						

COMMENTS:

DAILY TOTALS

Calories

Fat

Protein

Carbohydrates

Fiber

Other

Exercise and Fitness

DAILY PHYSICAL ACTIVITIES

ACTIVITY/ EXERCISE	hrs./ mins.	reps./ sets	------INTENSITY------ low	med	high	cal. burned
TOTAL CALORIES BURNED						

COMMENTS:

VITAMINS &
SUPPLEMENTS

Type:

Qty:

Type:

Qty:

Type:

Qty:

Type:

Qty:

Type:

Qty:

Type:

Qty:

Daily Assessment and Notes

OBSTACLES, SOLUTIONS AND THOUGHTS ON YOUR PROGRESS

WEIGHT

Helpful Tips
for Effective
Weight-Loss

If you're traveling
and away from
your gym, use the
stairs and walk as
much as possible,
or try to book a
hotel room with a
fitness facility.

Daily Nutritional Intake

FOOD AND BEVERAGES

MORNING TIME:	amt.	cal.	fat gms	protein gms	carbs. gms	fiber gms
BREAKFAST TOTALS						

COMMENTS:

AFTERNOON TIME:	amt.	cal.	fat gms	protein gms	carbs. gms	fiber gms
LUNCH TOTALS						

COMMENTS:

Daily Serving Intake

_____ Fruits
# of servings

_____ Vegetables
# of servings

_____ Grains
# of servings

_____ Meat & Beans
# of servings

_____ Milk & Dairy
# of servings

_____ Oils & Sweets
# of servings

EVENING TIME:	amt.	cal.	fat gms	protein gms	carbs. gms	fiber gms
DINNER TOTALS						

Water Intake

oz.

COMMENTS:

Daily Nutritional Intake

FOOD AND BEVERAGES

**DAILY GOALS
ACHIEVED**

SNACKS TIME:	amt.	cal.	fat gms	protein gms	carbs. gms	fiber gms
SNACK TOTALS						

COMMENTS:

DAILY TOTALS

Calories

Fat

Protein

Carbohydrates

Fiber

Other

Exercise and Fitness

DAILY PHYSICAL ACTIVITIES

ACTIVITY/ EXERCISE	hrs./ mins.	reps./ sets	low	med	high	cal. burned
TOTAL CALORIES BURNED						

------INTENSITY------

COMMENTS:

**VITAMINS &
SUPPLEMENTS**

Type:
Qty:
Type:
Qty:
Type:
Qty:
Type:
Qty:
Type:
Qty:
Type:
Qty:

Daily Assessment and Notes

OBSTACLES, SOLUTIONS AND THOUGHTS ON YOUR PROGRESS

**Helpful Tips
for Effective
Weight-Loss**

Increase the
intensity of your
workouts only
when your body is
ready. Trying to
force too much, too
soon can potential-
ly harm you and
your body.

Daily Nutritional Intake

FOOD AND BEVERAGES

MORNING TIME:	amt.	cal.	fat gms	protein gms	carbs. gms	fiber gms
BREAKFAST TOTALS						

COMMENTS:

AFTERNOON TIME:	amt.	cal.	fat gms	protein gms	carbs. gms	fiber gms
LUNCH TOTALS						

COMMENTS:

Daily Serving Intake

_____ Fruits
# of servings

_____ Vegetables
# of servings

_____ Grains
# of servings

_____ Meat & Beans
# of servings

_____ Milk & Dairy
# of servings

_____ Oils & Sweets
# of servings

EVENING TIME:	amt.	cal.	fat gms	protein gms	carbs. gms	fiber gms
DINNER TOTALS						

COMMENTS:

Water Intake

oz. _____

☐ low   ☐ med   ☐ high

ENERGY LEVELS

Daily Nutritional Intake

FOOD AND BEVERAGES

**DAILY GOALS
ACHIEVED**

SNACKS TIME:	amt.	cal.	fat gms	protein gms	carbs. gms	fiber gms
SNACK TOTALS						

COMMENTS:

DAILY TOTALS

Calories

Fat

Protein

Carbohydrates

Fiber

Other

Exercise and Fitness

DAILY PHYSICAL ACTIVITIES

ACTIVITY/ EXERCISE	hrs./ mins.	reps./ sets	low	med	high	cal. burned
TOTAL CALORIES BURNED						

------INTENSITY------

COMMENTS:

**VITAMINS &
SUPPLEMENTS**

Type:

Qty:

Type:

Qty:

Type:

Qty:

Type:

Qty:

Type:

Qty:

Type:

Qty:

Daily Assessment and Notes

OBSTACLES, SOLUTIONS AND THOUGHTS ON YOUR PROGRESS

DATE

WEIGHT

Helpful Tips
for Effective
Weight-Loss

Work out because
you want to. Make
it the time of day
when it's all about
you.

Daily Nutritional Intake

FOOD AND BEVERAGES

MORNING TIME:	amt.	cal.	fat gms	protein gms	carbs. gms	fiber gms
BREAKFAST TOTALS						

COMMENTS:

AFTERNOON TIME:	amt.	cal.	fat gms	protein gms	carbs. gms	fiber gms
LUNCH TOTALS						

COMMENTS:

Daily Serving Intake

_____ Fruits
# of servings

_____ Vegetables
# of servings

_____ Grains
# of servings

_____ Meat & Beans
# of servings

_____ Milk & Dairy
# of servings

_____ Oils & Sweets
# of servings

EVENING TIME:	amt.	cal.	fat gms	protein gms	carbs. gms	fiber gms
DINNER TOTALS						

Water Intake

oz.

COMMENTS:

❏ low ❏ med ❏ high

ENERGY LEVELS

Daily Nutritional Intake

FOOD AND BEVERAGES

**DAILY GOALS
ACHIEVED**

DAILY TOTALS

SNACKS TIME:	amt.	cal.	fat gms	protein gms	carbs. gms	fiber gms
SNACK TOTALS						

COMMENTS:

Calories

Fat

Protein

Carbohydrates

Fiber

Other

Exercise and Fitness

DAILY PHYSICAL ACTIVITIES

**VITAMINS &
SUPPLEMENTS**

ACTIVITY/ EXERCISE	hrs./ mins.	reps./ sets	INTENSITY low	med	high	cal. burned
TOTAL CALORIES BURNED						

COMMENTS:

Type:
Qty:
Type:
Qty:
Type:
Qty:
Type:
Qty:
Type:
Qty:
Type:
Qty:

Daily Assessment and Notes

OBSTACLES, SOLUTIONS AND THOUGHTS ON YOUR PROGRESS

Daily Nutritional Intake

FOOD AND BEVERAGES

MORNING TIME:	amt.	cal.	fat gms	protein gms	carbs. gms	fiber gms
BREAKFAST TOTALS						

COMMENTS:

AFTERNOON TIME:	amt.	cal.	fat gms	protein gms	carbs. gms	fiber gms
LUNCH TOTALS						

COMMENTS:

EVENING TIME:	amt.	cal.	fat gms	protein gms	carbs. gms	fiber gms
DINNER TOTALS						

COMMENTS:

Daily Serving Intake

_____ Fruits
# of servings

_____ Vegetables
# of servings

_____ Grains
# of servings

_____ Meat & Beans
# of servings

_____ Milk & Dairy
# of servings

_____ Oils & Sweets
# of servings

Water Intake

oz. _____

☐ low   ☐ med   ☐ high

ENERGY LEVELS

Daily Nutritional Intake

FOOD AND BEVERAGES

SNACKS TIME:	amt.	cal.	fat gms	protein gms	carbs. gms	fiber gms
SNACK TOTALS						

COMMENTS:

DAILY TOTALS

Calories

Fat

Protein

Carbohydrates

Fiber

Other

Exercise and Fitness

DAILY PHYSICAL ACTIVITIES

ACTIVITY/ EXERCISE	hrs./ mins.	reps./ sets	------INTENSITY------ low	med	high	cal. burned
TOTAL CALORIES BURNED						

COMMENTS:

VITAMINS &
SUPPLEMENTS

Type:
Qty:
Type:
Qty:
Type:
Qty:
Type:
Qty:
Type:
Qty:
Type:
Qty:

Daily Assessment and Notes

OBSTACLES, SOLUTIONS AND THOUGHTS ON YOUR PROGRESS

WEIGHT

Daily Nutritional Intake

FOOD AND BEVERAGES

MORNING TIME:	amt.	cal.	fat gms	protein gms	carbs. gms	fiber gms
BREAKFAST TOTALS						

COMMENTS:

AFTERNOON TIME:	amt.	cal.	fat gms	protein gms	carbs. gms	fiber gms
LUNCH TOTALS						

COMMENTS:

Daily Serving Intake

_____ Fruits
# of servings

_____ Vegetables
# of servings

_____ Grains
# of servings

_____ Meat & Beans
# of servings

_____ Milk & Dairy
# of servings

_____ Oils & Sweets
# of servings

EVENING TIME:	amt.	cal.	fat gms	protein gms	carbs. gms	fiber gms
DINNER TOTALS						

Water Intake

oz.

COMMENTS:

□ low   □ med   □ high

ENERGY LEVELS

Daily Nutritional Intake

FOOD AND BEVERAGES

DAILY GOALS
ACHIEVED

SNACKS TIME:	amt.	cal.	fat gms	protein gms	carbs. gms	fiber gms
SNACK TOTALS						

COMMENTS:

DAILY TOTALS

Calories

Fat

Protein

Carbohydrates

Fiber

Other

Exercise and Fitness

DAILY PHYSICAL ACTIVITIES

ACTIVITY/ EXERCISE	hrs./ mins.	reps./ sets	low	med	high	cal. burned
TOTAL CALORIES BURNED						

------INTENSITY------

COMMENTS:

VITAMINS &
SUPPLEMENTS

Type:
Qty:
Type:
Qty:
Type:
Qty:
Type:
Qty:
Type:
Qty:
Type:
Qty:

Daily Assessment and Notes

OBSTACLES, SOLUTIONS AND THOUGHTS ON YOUR PROGRESS

WEIGHT

Helpful Tips
for Effective
Weight-Loss

Daily Nutritional Intake

FOOD AND BEVERAGES

Before you begin
eating, determine
how much food on
your plate you are
going to eat. Doing
this will help you
keep your portion
sizes sensible and
prevent you from
overeating.

MORNING TIME:	amt.	cal.	fat gms	protein gms	carbs. gms	fiber gms
BREAKFAST TOTALS						

COMMENTS:

AFTERNOON TIME:	amt.	cal.	fat gms	protein gms	carbs. gms	fiber gms
LUNCH TOTALS						

COMMENTS:

Daily Serving Intake

____ Fruits
# of servings

____ Vegetables
# of servings

____ Grains
# of servings

____ Meat & Beans
# of servings

____ Milk & Dairy
# of servings

____ Oils & Sweets
# of servings

Water Intake

oz.

EVENING TIME:	amt.	cal.	fat gms	protein gms	carbs. gms	fiber gms
DINNER TOTALS						

COMMENTS:

☐ low   ☐ med   ☐ high

ENERGY LEVELS

Daily Nutritional Intake

FOOD AND BEVERAGES

DAILY GOALS
ACHIEVED

SNACKS TIME:	amt.	cal.	fat gms	protein gms	carbs. gms	fiber gms
SNACK TOTALS						

COMMENTS:

DAILY TOTALS

Calories

Fat

Protein

Carbohydrates

Fiber

Other

Exercise and Fitness

DAILY PHYSICAL ACTIVITIES

ACTIVITY/ EXERCISE	hrs./ mins.	reps./ sets	------INTENSITY------ low	med	high	cal. burned
TOTAL CALORIES BURNED						

COMMENTS:

VITAMINS &
SUPPLEMENTS

Type:

Qty:

Type:

Qty:

Type:

Qty:

Type:

Qty:

Type:

Qty:

Type:

Qty:

Daily Assessment and Notes

OBSTACLES, SOLUTIONS AND THOUGHTS ON YOUR PROGRESS

**Helpful Tips
for Effective
Weight-Loss**

Take each day of
your weight-loss
program one day at
a time.

Daily Nutritional Intake

FOOD AND BEVERAGES

MORNING TIME:	amt.	cal.	fat gms	protein gms	carbs. gms	fiber gms
BREAKFAST TOTALS						

COMMENTS:

AFTERNOON TIME:	amt.	cal.	fat gms	protein gms	carbs. gms	fiber gms
LUNCH TOTALS						

COMMENTS:

Daily Serving Intake

____ Fruits
# of servings

____ Vegetables
# of servings

____ Grains
# of servings

____ Meat & Beans
# of servings

____ Milk & Dairy
# of servings

____ Oils & Sweets
# of servings

EVENING TIME:	amt.	cal.	fat gms	protein gms	carbs. gms	fiber gms
DINNER TOTALS						

COMMENTS:

Water Intake

oz. _____

□ low □ med □ high

ENERGY LEVELS

Daily Nutritional Intake

FOOD AND BEVERAGES

DAILY GOALS
ACHIEVED

DAILY TOTALS

SNACKS TIME:	amt.	cal.	fat gms	protein gms	carbs. gms	fiber gms
SNACK TOTALS						

COMMENTS:

Calories

Fat

Protein

Carbohydrates

Fiber

Other

Exercise and Fitness

DAILY PHYSICAL ACTIVITIES

VITAMINS &
SUPPLEMENTS

ACTIVITY/ EXERCISE	hrs./ mins.	reps./ sets	------INTENSITY------ low	med	high	cal. burned
TOTAL CALORIES BURNED						

COMMENTS:

Type:

Qty:

Type:

Qty:

Type:

Qty:

Type:

Qty:

Type:

Qty:

Type:

Qty:

Daily Assessment and Notes

OBSTACLES, SOLUTIONS AND THOUGHTS ON YOUR PROGRESS

WEIGHT

Daily Nutritional Intake

FOOD AND BEVERAGES

MORNING TIME:	amt.	cal.	fat gms	protein gms	carbs. gms	fiber gms
BREAKFAST TOTALS						

COMMENTS:

AFTERNOON TIME:	amt.	cal.	fat gms	protein gms	carbs. gms	fiber gms
LUNCH TOTALS						

COMMENTS:

Daily Serving Intake

____ Fruits
       # of servings

____ Vegetables
       # of servings

____ Grains
       # of servings

____ Meat & Beans
       # of servings

____ Milk & Dairy
       # of servings

____ Oils & Sweets
       # of servings

Water Intake

oz.

EVENING TIME:	amt.	cal.	fat gms	protein gms	carbs. gms	fiber gms
DINNER TOTALS						

COMMENTS:

Daily Nutritional Intake

FOOD AND BEVERAGES

**DAILY GOALS
ACHIEVED**

DAILY TOTALS

SNACKS TIME:	amt.	cal.	fat gms	protein gms	carbs. gms	fiber gms
SNACK TOTALS						

COMMENTS:

Calories

Fat

Protein

Carbohydrates

Fiber

Other

Exercise and Fitness

DAILY PHYSICAL ACTIVITIES

**VITAMINS &
SUPPLEMENTS**

ACTIVITY/ EXERCISE	hrs./ mins.	reps./ sets	low	med	high	cal. burned
TOTAL CALORIES BURNED						

INTENSITY

COMMENTS:

Type:

Qty:

Type:

Qty:

Type:

Qty:

Type:

Qty:

Type:

Qty:

Type:

Qty:

Daily Assessment and Notes

OBSTACLES, SOLUTIONS AND THOUGHTS ON YOUR PROGRESS

_____

_____

_____

_____

_____

Helpful Tips for Effective Weight-Loss

Incorporate all aspects of your weight-loss program into your daily routine. This way, instead of automatically reaching for a bag of chips, you will reach for a piece of fruit.

Daily Nutritional Intake

FOOD AND BEVERAGES

MORNING TIME:	amt.	cal.	fat gms	protein gms	carbs. gms	fiber gms
BREAKFAST TOTALS						

COMMENTS:

AFTERNOON TIME:	amt.	cal.	fat gms	protein gms	carbs. gms	fiber gms
LUNCH TOTALS						

COMMENTS:

EVENING TIME:	amt.	cal.	fat gms	protein gms	carbs. gms	fiber gms
DINNER TOTALS						

COMMENTS:

Daily Serving Intake

_____ Fruits
# of servings

_____ Vegetables
# of servings

_____ Grains
# of servings

_____ Meat & Beans
# of servings

_____ Milk & Dairy
# of servings

_____ Oils & Sweets
# of servings

Water Intake

oz.

☐ low ☐ med ☐ high

ENERGY LEVELS

**DAILY GOALS
ACHIEVED**

Daily Nutritional Intake

FOOD AND BEVERAGES

DAILY TOTALS

SNACKS TIME:	amt.	cal.	fat gms	protein gms	carbs. gms	fiber gms
SNACK TOTALS						

COMMENTS:

Calories

Fat

Protein

Carbohydrates

Fiber

Other

Exercise and Fitness

DAILY PHYSICAL ACTIVITIES

VITAMINS &
SUPPLEMENTS

ACTIVITY/ EXERCISE	hrs./ mins.	reps./ sets	------INTENSITY------ low	med	high	cal. burned
TOTAL CALORIES BURNED						

COMMENTS:

Type:
Qty:
Type:
Qty:
Type:
Qty:
Type:
Qty:
Type:
Qty:
Type:
Qty:

Daily Assessment and Notes

OBSTACLES, SOLUTIONS AND THOUGHTS ON YOUR PROGRESS

Daily Nutritional Intake

FOOD AND BEVERAGES

Helpful Tips
for Effective
Weight-Loss

Choose your diet
plan carefully.
You won't stick to
a diet with foods
you don't like, so
choose a program
that will include
your favorite foods.

MORNING TIME:	amt.	cal.	fat gms	protein gms	carbs. gms	fiber gms
BREAKFAST TOTALS						

COMMENTS:

AFTERNOON TIME:	amt.	cal.	fat gms	protein gms	carbs. gms	fiber gms
LUNCH TOTALS						

COMMENTS:

Daily Serving Intake

____ Fruits
# of servings

____ Vegetables
# of servings

____ Grains
# of servings

____ Meat & Beans
# of servings

____ Milk & Dairy
# of servings

____ Oils & Sweets
# of servings

EVENING TIME:	amt.	cal.	fat gms	protein gms	carbs. gms	fiber gms
DINNER TOTALS						

Water Intake

oz.

COMMENTS:

Daily Nutritional Intake

FOOD AND BEVERAGES

DAILY GOALS
ACHIEVED

SNACKS TIME:	amt.	cal.	fat gms	protein gms	carbs. gms	fiber gms
SNACK TOTALS						

COMMENTS:

DAILY TOTALS

Calories

Fat

Protein

Carbohydrates

Fiber

Other

Exercise and Fitness

DAILY PHYSICAL ACTIVITIES

ACTIVITY/ EXERCISE	hrs./ mins.	reps./ sets	------INTENSITY------ low	med	high	cal. burned
TOTAL CALORIES BURNED						

COMMENTS:

VITAMINS & SUPPLEMENTS

Type:
Qty:
Type:
Qty:
Type:
Qty:
Type:
Qty:
Type:
Qty:
Type:
Qty:

Daily Assessment and Notes

OBSTACLES, SOLUTIONS AND THOUGHTS ON YOUR PROGRESS

WEIGHT

Daily Nutritional Intake

FOOD AND BEVERAGES

Instead of choosing
pie or cake for
dessert, choose a
piece of fruit or
fruit-based fare.
Fruit can be more
refreshing than
sweets, and will
still satisfy your
sweet tooth.

MORNING TIME:	amt.	cal.	fat gms	protein gms	carbs. gms	fiber gms
		·				
BREAKFAST TOTALS						

COMMENTS:

AFTERNOON TIME:	amt.	cal.	fat gms	protein gms	carbs. gms	fiber gms
LUNCH TOTALS						

COMMENTS:

Daily Serving Intake

____ Fruits
# of servings

____ Vegetables
# of servings

____ Grains
# of servings

____ Meat & Beans
# of servings

____ Milk & Dairy
# of servings

____ Oils & Sweets
# of servings

Water Intake

oz.

EVENING TIME:	amt.	cal.	fat gms	protein gms	carbs. gms	fiber gms
DINNER TOTALS						

COMMENTS:

Daily Nutritional Intake

FOOD AND BEVERAGES

DAILY GOALS
ACHIEVED

SNACKS TIME:	amt.	cal.	fat gms	protein gms	carbs. gms	fiber gms
SNACK TOTALS						

COMMENTS:

DAILY TOTALS

Calories

Fat

Protein

Carbohydrates

Fiber

Other

Exercise and Fitness

DAILY PHYSICAL ACTIVITIES

ACTIVITY/ EXERCISE	hrs./ mins.	reps./ sets	INTENSITY low	med	high	cal. burned
TOTAL CALORIES BURNED						

COMMENTS:

VITAMINS &

SUPPLEMENTS

Type:

Qty:

Type:

Qty:

Type:

Qty:

Type:

Qty:

Type:

Qty:

Type:

Qty:

Daily Assessment and Notes

OBSTACLES, SOLUTIONS AND THOUGHTS ON YOUR PROGRESS

Make healthy
substitutions when
cooking a meal.
For example, use 2
egg whites instead
of 1 egg, or replace
the oil in a recipe
with applesauce.

Daily Nutritional Intake

FOOD AND BEVERAGES

MORNING TIME:	amt.	cal.	fat gms	protein gms	carbs. gms	fiber gms
BREAKFAST TOTALS						

COMMENTS:

AFTERNOON TIME:	amt.	cal.	fat gms	protein gms	carbs. gms	fiber gms
LUNCH TOTALS						

COMMENTS:

Daily Serving Intake

____ Fruits
# of servings

____ Vegetables
# of servings

____ Grains
# of servings

____ Meat & Beans
# of servings

____ Milk & Dairy
# of servings

____ Oils & Sweets
# of servings

EVENING TIME:	amt.	cal.	fat gms	protein gms	carbs. gms	fiber gms
DINNER TOTALS						

COMMENTS:

Water Intake

oz.

❏ low ❏ med ❏ high

ENERGY LEVELS

Daily Nutritional Intake

FOOD AND BEVERAGES

DAILY GOALS
ACHIEVED

SNACKS TIME:	amt.	cal.	fat gms	protein gms	carbs. gms	fiber gms
SNACK TOTALS						

COMMENTS:

DAILY TOTALS

Calories

Fat

Protein

Carbohydrates

Fiber

Other

Exercise and Fitness

DAILY PHYSICAL ACTIVITIES

ACTIVITY/ EXERCISE	hrs./ mins.	reps./ sets	------INTENSITY------			cal. burned
			low	med	high	
TOTAL CALORIES BURNED						

COMMENTS:

VITAMINS &
SUPPLEMENTS

Type:
Qty:
Type:
Qty:
Type:
Qty:
Type:
Qty:
Type:
Qty:
Type:
Qty:
Type:
Qty:

Daily Assessment and Notes

OBSTACLES, SOLUTIONS AND THOUGHTS ON YOUR PROGRESS

WEIGHT

Daily Nutritional Intake

FOOD AND BEVERAGES

A good incentive to
lose weight may be
all you need to get
started.

Write down the
reasons why you
want to lose
weight, and review
them each week to
keep up your
motivation.

MORNING TIME:		amt.	cal.	fat gms	protein gms	carbs. gms	fiber gms
BREAKFAST TOTALS							

COMMENTS:

AFTERNOON TIME:		amt.	cal.	fat gms	protein gms	carbs. gms	fiber gms
LUNCH TOTALS							

COMMENTS:

Daily Serving Intake

_____ Fruits
# of servings

_____ Vegetables
# of servings

_____ Grains
# of servings

_____ Meat & Beans
# of servings

_____ Milk & Dairy
# of servings

_____ Oils & Sweets
# of servings

EVENING TIME:		amt.	cal.	fat gms	protein gms	carbs. gms	fiber gms
DINNER TOTALS							

COMMENTS:

Water Intake

oz.

Daily Nutritional Intake

FOOD AND BEVERAGES

DAILY GOALS
ACHIEVED

SNACKS TIME:	amt.	cal.	fat gms	protein gms	carbs. gms	fiber gms
SNACK TOTALS						

COMMENTS:

DAILY TOTALS

Calories

Fat

Protein

Carbohydrates

Fiber

Other

Exercise and Fitness

DAILY PHYSICAL ACTIVITIES

ACTIVITY/ EXERCISE	hrs./ mins.	reps./ sets	low	med	high	cal. burned
TOTAL CALORIES BURNED						

(INTENSITY spans low / med / high columns)

COMMENTS:

VITAMINS &
SUPPLEMENTS

Type:
Qty:
Type:
Qty:
Type:
Qty:
Type:
Qty:
Type:
Qty:
Type:
Qty:

Daily Assessment and Notes

OBSTACLES, SOLUTIONS AND THOUGHTS ON YOUR PROGRESS

DATE

WEIGHT

Helpful Tips
for Effective
Weight-Loss

Let your friends
and family know
that you are dieting
so they can offer
support and
encouragement.
Having this kind of
support can also
help keep you
accountable for
your weight-loss
program.

Daily Nutritional Intake

FOOD AND BEVERAGES

MORNING TIME:		amt.	cal.	fat gms	protein gms	carbs. gms	fiber gms
BREAKFAST TOTALS							

COMMENTS:

AFTERNOON TIME:		amt.	cal.	fat gms	protein gms	carbs. gms	fiber gms
LUNCH TOTALS							

COMMENTS:

EVENING TIME:		amt.	cal.	fat gms	protein gms	carbs. gms	fiber gms
DINNER TOTALS							

COMMENTS:

Daily Serving Intake

_____ Fruits
# of servings

_____ Vegetables
# of servings

_____ Grains
# of servings

_____ Meat & Beans
# of servings

_____ Milk & Dairy
# of servings

_____ Oils & Sweets
# of servings

Water Intake

oz.

☐ low ☐ med ☐ high

ENERGY LEVELS

Daily Nutritional Intake

FOOD AND BEVERAGES

DAILY GOALS ACHIEVED

DAILY TOTALS

SNACKS TIME:	amt.	cal.	fat gms	protein gms	carbs. gms	fiber gms
SNACK TOTALS						

COMMENTS:

Calories

Fat

Protein

Carbohydrates

Fiber

Other

Exercise and Fitness

DAILY PHYSICAL ACTIVITIES

VITAMINS & SUPPLEMENTS

ACTIVITY/ EXERCISE	hrs./ mins.	reps./ sets	------INTENSITY------ low	med	high	cal. burned
TOTAL CALORIES BURNED						

COMMENTS:

Type:
Qty:
Type:
Qty:
Type:
Qty:
Type:
Qty:
Type:
Qty:
Type:
Qty:

Daily Assessment and Notes

OBSTACLES, SOLUTIONS AND THOUGHTS ON YOUR PROGRESS

DATE   WEIGHT

Helpful Tips for Effective Weight-Loss

Instead of coffee in the morning, try switching to green tea. Studies have shown a possible correlation between antioxidants found in green tea and overall good health.

With only 1/3 to 1/2 the caffeine as coffee per cup, green tea will give you a boost, but will less likely keep you up at night.

Daily Serving Intake

____ Fruits
# of servings

____ Vegetables
# of servings

____ Grains
# of servings

____ Meat & Beans
# of servings

____ Milk & Dairy
# of servings

____ Oils & Sweets
# of servings

Water Intake

oz.

Daily Nutritional Intake

FOOD AND BEVERAGES

MORNING TIME:	amt.	cal.	fat gms	protein gms	carbs. gms	fiber gms
BREAKFAST TOTALS						

COMMENTS:

AFTERNOON TIME:	amt.	cal.	fat gms	protein gms	carbs. gms	fiber gms
LUNCH TOTALS						

COMMENTS:

EVENING TIME:	amt.	cal.	fat gms	protein gms	carbs. gms	fiber gms
DINNER TOTALS						

COMMENTS:

☐ low ☐ med ☐ high

ENERGY LEVELS

Daily Nutritional Intake

FOOD AND BEVERAGES

**DAILY GOALS
ACHIEVED**

DAILY TOTALS

SNACKS TIME:	amt.	cal.	fat gms	protein gms	carbs. gms	fiber gms
SNACK TOTALS						

COMMENTS:

Calories

Fat

Protein

Carbohydrates

Fiber

Other

Exercise and Fitness

DAILY PHYSICAL ACTIVITIES

**VITAMINS &
SUPPLEMENTS**

ACTIVITY/ EXERCISE	hrs./ mins.	reps./ sets	low	med	high	cal. burned
TOTAL CALORIES BURNED						

(header spanning low/med/high: ------INTENSITY------)

COMMENTS:

Type:
Qty:
Type:
Qty:
Type:
Qty:
Type:
Qty:
Type:
Qty:
Type:
Qty:

Daily Assessment and Notes

OBSTACLES, SOLUTIONS AND THOUGHTS ON YOUR PROGRESS

Helpful Tips
for Effective
Weight-Loss

Try to set a time, preferably a few hours before you go to bed, to stop eating for the day. If you have to have a late-night snack, make it something sensible, like trail mix or fruit.

Daily Nutritional Intake

FOOD AND BEVERAGES

MORNING TIME:	amt.	cal.	fat gms	protein gms	carbs. gms	fiber gms
BREAKFAST TOTALS						

COMMENTS:

AFTERNOON TIME:	amt.	cal.	fat gms	protein gms	carbs. gms	fiber gms
LUNCH TOTALS						

COMMENTS:

Daily Serving Intake

_____ Fruits
# of servings

_____ Vegetables
# of servings

_____ Grains
# of servings

_____ Meat & Beans
# of servings

_____ Milk & Dairy
# of servings

_____ Oils & Sweets
# of servings

EVENING TIME:	amt.	cal.	fat gms	protein gms	carbs. gms	fiber gms
DINNER TOTALS						

COMMENTS:

Water Intake

oz. _____

**DAILY GOALS
ACHIEVED**

Daily Nutritional Intake

FOOD AND BEVERAGES

DAILY TOTALS

SNACKS TIME:	amt.	cal.	fat gms	protein gms	carbs. gms	fiber gms
SNACK TOTALS						

COMMENTS:

Calories

Fat

Protein

Carbohydrates

Fiber

Other

Exercise and Fitness

DAILY PHYSICAL ACTIVITIES

**VITAMINS &
SUPPLEMENTS**

ACTIVITY/ EXERCISE	hrs./ mins.	reps./ sets	------INTENSITY------ low	med	high	cal. burned
TOTAL CALORIES BURNED						

COMMENTS:

Type:

Qty:

Type:

Qty:

Type:

Qty:

Type:

Qty:

Type:

Qty:

Type:

Qty:

Daily Assessment and Notes

OBSTACLES, SOLUTIONS AND THOUGHTS ON YOUR PROGRESS

Daily Nutritional Intake

FOOD AND BEVERAGES

MORNING TIME:		amt.	cal.	fat gms	protein gms	carbs. gms	fiber gms
BREAKFAST TOTALS							

COMMENTS:

AFTERNOON TIME:		amt.	cal.	fat gms	protein gms	carbs. gms	fiber gms
LUNCH TOTALS							

COMMENTS:

EVENING TIME:		amt.	cal.	fat gms	protein gms	carbs. gms	fiber gms
DINNER TOTALS							

COMMENTS:

Daily Serving Intake

_____ Fruits
# of servings

_____ Vegetables
# of servings

_____ Grains
# of servings

_____ Meat & Beans
# of servings

_____ Milk & Dairy
# of servings

_____ Oils & Sweets
# of servings

Water Intake

oz.

Daily Nutritional Intake

FOOD AND BEVERAGES

DAILY GOALS
ACHIEVED

SNACKS TIME:		amt.	cal.	fat gms	protein gms	carbs. gms	fiber gms
SNACK TOTALS							

COMMENTS:

DAILY TOTALS

Calories

Fat

Protein

Carbohydrates

Fiber

Other

Exercise and Fitness

DAILY PHYSICAL ACTIVITIES

ACTIVITY/ EXERCISE	hrs./ mins.	reps./ sets	------INTENSITY------ low	med	high	cal. burned
TOTAL CALORIES BURNED						

COMMENTS:

VITAMINS &

SUPPLEMENTS

Type:

Qty:

Type:

Qty:

Type:

Qty:

Type:

Qty:

Type:

Qty:

Type:

Qty:

Daily Assessment and Notes

OBSTACLES, SOLUTIONS AND THOUGHTS ON YOUR PROGRESS

Daily Nutritional Intake

FOOD AND BEVERAGES

MORNING TIME:	amt.	cal.	fat gms	protein gms	carbs. gms	fiber gms
BREAKFAST TOTALS						

COMMENTS:

AFTERNOON TIME:	amt.	cal.	fat gms	protein gms	carbs. gms	fiber gms
LUNCH TOTALS						

COMMENTS:

Daily Serving Intake

_____ Fruits
# of servings

_____ Vegetables
# of servings

_____ Grains
# of servings

_____ Meat & Beans
# of servings

_____ Milk & Dairy
# of servings

_____ Oils & Sweets
# of servings

EVENING TIME:	amt.	cal.	fat gms	protein gms	carbs. gms	fiber gms
DINNER TOTALS						

Water Intake

oz.

COMMENTS:

❏ low   ❏ med   ❏ high

ENERGY LEVELS

Daily Nutritional Intake

FOOD AND BEVERAGES

DAILY GOALS ACHIEVED

DAILY TOTALS

SNACKS TIME:	amt.	cal.	fat gms	protein gms	carbs. gms	fiber gms
SNACK TOTALS						

COMMENTS:

Calories

Fat

Protein

Carbohydrates

Fiber

Other

Exercise and Fitness

DAILY PHYSICAL ACTIVITIES

VITAMINS &

SUPPLEMENTS

ACTIVITY/ EXERCISE	hrs./ mins.	reps./ sets	------INTENSITY------			cal. burned
			low	med	high	
TOTAL CALORIES BURNED						

COMMENTS:

Type:

Qty:

Type:

Qty:

Type:

Qty:

Type:

Qty:

Type:

Qty:

Type:

Qty:

Daily Assessment and Notes

OBSTACLES, SOLUTIONS AND THOUGHTS ON YOUR PROGRESS

NOTES

NUTRITIONAL FACTS ON POPULAR FOOD ITEMS

This section is a great resource for nutritional information on foods you may want to select for your weight-loss program. It will provide calories per serving, as well as the content in grams for protein, fats, carbohydrates, and fiber.

To use this section, look up food items which are listed in alphabetical order. Locate the corresponding information, and log the data into your journal so you can track your daily totals.

NUTRITIONAL INFORMATION

Nutrition values for fat, protein, carbohydrates, and fiber are listed in grams per serving.
Serving sizes and values are approximate.

FOOD ITEM	Serving Size	Cal.	Fat	Protein	Carbs	Fiber
A						
Alcohol, 100 proof	1 fl oz	82	0	0	0	0
Alcohol, 86 proof	1 fl oz	70	0	0	0	0
Alcohol, 90 proof	1 fl oz	73	0	0	0	0
Alcohol, 94 proof	1 fl oz	76	0	0	0	0
Alcohol, dessert wine, dry	1 glass	157	0	0.2	12	0
Alcohol, dessert wine, sweet	1 glass	165	0	0.2	14.1	0
Alcohol, liquors	1 fl oz	107	0.1	0	11.2	0
Alcohol, pina colada	8 fl oz	440	4.8	1	57	0.4
Alfalfa seeds	1 tbsp	1	0	0.1	0.1	0.1
Allspice, ground	1 tsp	5	0.2	0.1	1.4	0.4
Almond butter, w/ salt	1 tbsp	101	9.5	2.4	3.4	0.6
Almond butter, w/o salt	1 tbsp	101	9.5	2.4	3.4	0.6
Almonds, roasted	1 oz (12 nuts)	169	15	6.2	5.5	3.3
Anchovies	3 oz	111	4.1	17.3	0	0
Apple cider, powdered	1 packet	83	0	0	20.7	0
Apple juice	8 fl oz	120	0.2	0.2	28.8	0
Apples, w/o skin	1 medium	61	0.2	0.3	16	1.7
Apples, w/ skin	1 medium	72	0.2	0.4	19	3.3
Applesauce	1 cup	194	0.5	0.5	50.8	3.1
Apricots	1 apricot	17	0.1	0.5	3.9	0.7
Arrowroot	1 cup, sliced	78	0.2	5.1	16.1	1.6
Arrowroot flour	1 cup	457	0.1	0.4	112.8	4.4
Artichokes	1 artichoke	76	0.2	5.3	17	8.7
Arugula	1 cup	4	0.1	0.5	0.7	0.4
Asparagus	1 spear	2	0	0.3	0.5	0.3
Avocados	1 cup, cubes	240	22	3	12.8	10
B						
Bacon bits, meatless	1 tbsp	33	1.8	2.2	2	0.7
Bacon, canadian, cooked	1 slice	43	2	5.8	0.3	0
Bacon, meatless	1 slice	16	1.5	0.5	0.3	0.1
Bacon, pork, cooked	1 slice	42	3.2	3	0.1	0
Bagels, cinnamon-raisin	1 bagel, 4" dia	244	1.5	8.7	49	2
Bagels, egg	1 bagel, 4" dia	292	2.2	11	55.6	2.4
Bagels, oat-bran	1 bagel, 4" dia	227	1	9.5	47	3.2
Bagels, plain	1 bagel, 4" dia	245	1.4	9.3	47	2
Bagels, deli gourmet style	1 bagel	370	3	13	71	2
Balsam-pear	1 balsam-pear	21	0.2	1.2	4.6	3.5
Bamboo shoots	1 cup	41	0.5	3.9	7.9	3.3
Banana chips	1 oz	147	9.5	0.7	16.6	2.2
Bananas	1 medium, 7"-8"	105	0.4	13	27	3
Barley	1 cup	651	4.2	23	135.2	31.8
Barley flour	1 cup	511	2.4	15.5	110.3	14.9
Barley, pearled, cooked	1 cup	193	0.7	3.6	44.3	6
Basil	5 leaves	1	0	0.1	0.1	0.1
Basil, dried	1 tsp	2	0	0.1	0.4	0.3
Bay leaf	1 tsp, crumbled	2	0.1	0	0.4	0.2
Beans, adzuki, cooked	1 cup	294	0.2	17	57	16.8
Beans, baked, canned, plain	1 cup	239	0.9	12.1	53.7	10.4
Beans, baked, canned, w/o salt	1 cup	266	1	12.1	52.1	13.9

Nutrition values for fat, protein, carbohydrates, and fiber are listed in grams per serving.
Serving sizes and values are approximate.

FOOD ITEM	Serving Size	Cal.	Fat	Protein	Carbs	Fiber
B (cont.)						
Beans, baked, canned, w/ beef	1 cup	322	9.2	17	45	10
Beans, black, cooked	1 cup	227	0.9	15	40	15
Beans, cranberry, cooked	1 cup	241	0.8	16	43	18
Beans, fava, canned	1 cup	182	0.5	14	31	9.5
Beans, french, cooked	1 cup	228	1.3	12	43	17
Beans, great northern, cooked	1 cup	209	0.8	15	37	12
Beans, kidney, cooked	1 cup	225	0.9	15	40	11
Beans, lima, cooked	1 cup	216	0.7	15	39	13
Beans, lima, canned	1 can	190	0.4	12	36	11
Beans, mung, cooked	1 cup	212	0.7	14	39	15
Beans, mungo, cooked	1 cup	189	1	13.5	33	11.5
Beans, navy, cooked	1 cup	255	1	15	47	19
Beans, pink, cooked	1 cup	252	0.8	15	47	9
Beans, pinto, cooked	1 cup	245	1	15	44	15
Beans, small white, cooked	1 cup	254	1	16	46	18
Beans, snap, green, cooked	1 cup	44	0.3	2	10	4
Beans, snap, yellow, cooked	1 cup	44	0.3	2	10	4
Beans, white, cooked	1 cup	249	0.6	17	45	11
Beans, yellow	1 cup	255	2	16	48	18
Beechnuts, dried	1 oz	163	14.2	1.8	9.5	0
Beef ,choice short rib, cooked	3 oz	400	35.6	18.3	0	0
Beef bologna	1 slice	88	8	3.3	0.6	0
Beef jerky, chopped	1 piece	81	5.1	6.6	2.2	0.4
Beef sausage, pre-cooked	1 link	134	11.6	6	1	0
Beef stew, canned	1 serving	218	12.5	11.5	15.7	3.5
Beef, tri-tip roast, roasted	3 oz	174	9.4	22.2	0	0
Beef, brisket, lean and fat, roasted	3 oz	328	26.8	20	0	0
Beef, brisket, lean, roasted	3 oz	206	10.8	25.3	0	0
Beef, chuck ,arm roast, lean & fat, braised	3 oz	283	19.6	23.3	0	0
Beef, chuck ,arm roast, lean, braised	3 oz	179	6.5	28.1	0	0
Beef, chuck, top blade, raw	3 oz	138	7.5	16.5	0	0
Beef, cured breakfast strips	3 slices	276	26.4	8.5	0.5	0
Beef, cured, corned, canned	3 oz	213	12.8	23	0	0
Beef, cured, dried	1 serving	43	0.5	8.7	0.8	0
Beef, cured, luncheon meat	1 slice	31	0.9	5.4	0	0
Beef, flank, raw	1 oz	47	2.4	6	0	0
Beef, ground patties, frozen	3 oz	240	19.7	14.5	0	0
Beef, ground, 70% lean, raw	1 oz	94	8.5	4.1	0	0
Beef, ground, 80% lean, raw	1 oz	72	5.7	4.9	0	0
Beef, ground, 95% lean, raw	1 oz	39	1.4	6.1	0	0
Beef, rib, large end, boneless, raw	1 oz	94	8.3	4.5	0	0
Beef, rib, shortribs, boneless, raw	1 oz	110	10.3	4.1	0	0
Beef, rib, whole, boneless, raw	1 oz	91	7.9	4.6	0	0
Beef, rib-eye, small end, raw	1 oz	78	6.3	5	0	0
Beef, round, bottom, raw	1 oz	56	3.4	5.9	0	0
Beef, round, eye, raw	1 oz	49	2.5	6.1	0	0
Beef, round, full cut, raw	1 oz	55	3.4	5.8	0	0
Beef, round, tip, raw	1 oz	56	3.6	5.5	0	0
Beef, round, top, raw	1 oz	48	2.3	6.2	0	0
Beef, shank crosscuts, raw	1 oz	50	2.8	5.8	0	0

Nutrition values for fat, protein, carbohydrates, and fiber are listed in grams per serving.
Serving sizes and values are approximate.

FOOD ITEM	Serving Size	Cal.	Fat	Protein	Carbs	Fiber
B (cont.)						
Beef, short loin, porterhouse, raw	1 oz	73	5.7	5.1	0	0
Beef, short loin, t-bone, raw	1 oz	66	4.8	5.4	0	0
Beef, short loin, top, raw	1 oz	66	4.5	5.8	0	0
Beef, sirloin, tri-tip, raw	1 oz	50	3	5.8	0	0
Beef, tenderloin, raw	1 oz	70	5.1	5.6	0	0
Beef, top sirloin, raw	1 oz	61	4	5.6	0	0
Beer, light	12 fl oz.	110	12	4.8	7	0
Beer, non-alcoholic	12 fl oz.	80	1	0	70	0
Beer, regular	12 fl oz.	140	12	0.9	10	0.7
Beets	1 beet	35	0	2	8	4
Bratwurst, chicken	1 serving	148	8.7	16.3	0	0
Bratwurst, pork	1 serving	281	24.8	11.7	2.1	0
Bratwurst, veal	1 serving	286	26.6	11.8	0	0
Bread stuffing, dry mix, prepared	1/2 cup	178	8.6	3	22	3
Bread, banana	1 slice	196	6.3	2.5	32.7	0.7
Bread, corn	1 piece	188	6	4.3	28.8	1.4
Bread, cracked-wheat	1 slice	65	1	2.2	11.8	1
Bread, french	1 slice	70	1	3	15	1
Bread, garlic	1 slice	160	10	3	14	1
Bread, Irish soda	1 oz	82	1.4	1.9	15.9	0.7
Bread, pita	2 oz	150	1	3	30	0
Bread, pumpernickel	1 slice	75	1	3	15	2
Bread, raisin	1 slice	80	1.5	2	15	1
Bread, rice bran	1 oz	69	1.3	2.5	12.3	1.4
Bread, sandwich slice	1 slice	70	1	2	13	1
Bread, sourdough	1 slice	100	1	2	20	1
Broadbeans, cooked	1 cup	187	0.6	13	33.4	9.2
Brownies	1 brownie	220	13	1	27	1
Buckwheat	1 cup	583	5.8	22.5	121.6	17
Buckwheat flour	1 cup	402	3.7	15.1	84.7	12
Buckwheat groats, roasted, cooked	1 cup	155	1	5.6	33.5	4.5
Buffalo, raw	1 oz	28	0.4	5.8	0	0
Burbot, raw	3 oz	77	0.7	16.4	0	0
Burdock root	1 cup	85	0.2	1.8	20.5	3.9
Butter, whipped, w/ salt	1 tbsp	67	7.6	0.1	0	0
Butternuts, dried	1 oz	174	16	7	3	1.3
C						
Cabbage, common	1 cup, shredded	17	1	1	4	1.6
Cabbage, pak-choi	1 cup, shredded	9	0.1	1.1	1.5	0.7
Cabbage, pe-tsai	1 cup, shredded	12	0.2	0.9	2.5	0.9
Cake, angel food	1 slice	180	4	2	36	2
Cake, boston crème pie	1 slice	260	9	1	32	0
Cake, carrot	1 slice	310	16	1	39	0
Cake, cheesecake	1 slice	500	30	4	50	0
Cake, chocolate	1 slice	270	13	1	36	1
Cake, chocolate mousse	1 slice	250	10	1	35	1
Cake, devil's food	1 slice	270	13	2	35	0
Cake, pineapple upside-down	1 piece	367	13.9	4	58.1	0.9
Cake, pound	1 slice	320	16	2	38	0

NUTRITIONAL INFORMATION

Nutrition values for fat, protein, carbohydrates, and fiber are listed in grams per serving.
Serving sizes and values are approximate.

FOOD ITEM	Serving Size	Cal.	Fat	Protein	Carbs	Fiber
C (cont.)						
Cake, sponge cake w/ cream, berries	1 slice	325	8	25	38	1
Cake, yellow	1 slice	260	11	2	36	1
Candy, butterscotch	5 pieces	120	2.5	0	20	0
Candy, caramels	1 piece	30	1	3	6	1
Candy, carob	1 bar	470	27.3	7.1	49	3.3
Candy, chocolate fudge	1 oz.	125	5	0	18	0
Candy, chocolate mints	1 mint	45	1	0	9	0
Candy, milk chocolate w/ almonds	1.5 oz.	216	14	3.7	21	2.5
Candy, chocolate-coated peanut butter bites	1 piece	45	2.5	1	4	0
Candy, chocolate-coated peanuts	12 peanuts	160	11	20	15	7
Candy, gum drops	4 pieces	130	0	0	31	0
Candy, hard candy	1 piece	18	0	0	5	0
Candy, jellybeans	12 beans	100	0	0	24	0
Candy, licorice	1 piece	30	0	0	7	0
Candy, lollipop	1 lollipop	20	0	0	5	0
Candy, milk chocolate bar	1.5 oz.	235	13	3.3	26	1.5
Candy, mints	1 mint	30	0	0	7	0
Cantaloupe	1 cup, cubed	54	0.3	1.3	13.1	1.4
Cardoon	1 cup, shredded	36	0.2	1.2	8.7	2.8
Carrots	1 medium	65	0	1	15	4
Cashew butter, w/ salt	1 tbsp	94	7.9	2.8	4.4	0.3
Cashew nuts	1 oz.	157	12.4	5.2	8.6	0.9
Cassava	1 cup	330	0.6	2.8	78.4	3.7
Celeriac	1 cup	66	0.5	2.3	14.4	2.8
Chard, swiss	1 cup	7	0.1	0.6	1.3	0.6
Cheese, American	1 slice	110	9	5	1	0
Cheese, brick	1 oz.	100	8	31	0	0
Cheese, brie	1 oz.	95	8	50	1	0
Cheese, camembert	1 oz.	90	7	49	1	0
Cheese, cheddar	1 oz.	110	9	33	0.5	0
Cheese, colby-jack	1 oz.	110	9	31	0.5	0
Cheese, cottage, 2%	1 cup	203	4	31	8	0
Cheese, edam	1 oz.	100	8	7	0	0
Cheese, feta	1 oz.	100	8	21	1	0
Cheese, goat	1 oz	128	10.1	8.7	0.6	0
Cheese, goat, semi-soft	1 oz	103	8.5	6.1	0.7	0
Cheese, goat, soft	1 oz	76	6	5.3	0.3	0
Cheese, gouda	1 oz.	100	8	7	0.5	0
Cheese, monterey-jack	1 oz.	110	9	32	0	0
Cheese, mozzarella	1 oz.	90	7	25	0.5	0
Cheese, parmesan, hard	1 oz.	110	7	10	1	0
Cheese, parmesan, shredded	1 tbsp	22	1.5	2	0	0
Cheese, provolone	1 oz.	100	8	34	1	0
Cheese, queso	2 tbsp	110	9	28	2	0
Cheese, ricotta	2 tbsp	50	3.5	28	1	0
Cheese, roquefort	1 oz.	105	9	6	0.5	0
Cheese, swiss	1 oz.	110	9	36	1	0
Cherries, sour	8 pieces	30	0	1	7	2
Cherries, sweet	8 pieces	30	0	2	7	2
Chewing gum	1 piece	25	0	0	5	0

263

NUTRITIONAL INFORMATION

Nutrition values for fat, protein, carbohydrates, and fiber are listed in grams per serving.
Serving sizes and values are approximate.

FOOD ITEM	Serving Size	Cal.	Fat	Protein	Carbs	Fiber
C (cont.)						
Chicken, breast, w/ skin	1/2 breast	249	13.4	30.2	0	0
Chicken, breast, w/o skin	1/2 breast	130	1.5	27.2	0	0
Chicken, capons, boneless	1/2 capon	1459	74	184	0	0
Chicken, capons, giblets, cooked	1 cup	238	8	38	1	0
Chicken, cornish game hen, roasted	1/2 bird	336	24	29	0	0
Chicken, cornish game hen, meat only	1 bird	295	9	51	0	0
Chicken, dark meat, w/o skin	1 cup diced	287	14	38	0	0
Chicken, drumstick, w/ skin	1 drumstick	118	6.3	14.1	0	0
Chicken, drumstick, w/o skin	1 drumstick	74	2.1	12.8	0	0
Chicken, leg, w/ skin	1 leg	312	20.2	30.3	0	0
Chicken, leg, w/o skin	1 leg	156	5	26.2	0	0
Chicken, light meat, w/o skin	1 cup diced	214	6	38	0	0
Chicken, thigh, w/ skin	1 thigh	198	14.3	16.2	0	0
Chicken, thigh, w/o skin	1 thigh	82	2.7	13.6	0	0
Chicken, wing, w/ skin	1 wing	109	7.8	9	0	0
Chicken, wing, w/o skin	1 wing	37	1	6.4	0	0
Chickpeas, cooked	1 cup	269	4	15	45	12.5
Chicory greens	1 cup, chopped	41	0.5	3.1	8.5	7.2
Chicory roots	1/2 cup	33	0.1	0.6	7.9	0
Chicory, witloof	1/2 cup	8	0	0.4	1.8	1.4
Chili con carne w/ beans	1 cup	298	13	17.5	28	10
Chili powder	1 tsp	8	0.4	0.3	1.4	0.9
Chili w/ beans, canned	1 cup	287	14	14.5	30.5	11
Chili w/o beans, canned	1 cup	194	6.5	17	18	3
Chinese chestnuts	1 oz	64	0.3	1.2	13.9	0
Chives	1 tbsp, chopped	1	0	0.1	0.1	0.1
Chocolate chip crisped rice bar	1 bar	115	3.8	1.4	20.7	0.6
Chocolate chips	1/4 cup	210	12	3	24	1
Chocolate milkshake, ready-to-drink	8 fl oz	181	5	8	26	1
Chocolate, semi-sweet bars, baking	1 oz.	160	8	3	20	1
Chocolate, unsweetened baking squares	1 square	144	15	3.7	8.6	4.8
Chorizo, pork and beef	1 link	273	23	14.5	1.1	0
Chow mein noodles	1 cup	237	13.8	3.8	25.9	1.8
Cinnamon, ground	1 tsp	6	0.1	0.1	1.8	1.2
Cisco	3 oz	83	1.6	16.1	0	0
Citrus fruit drink, from concentrate	8 fl oz	124	0.1	0.5	30	0.8
Clam, mixed species, raw	1 large	15	0.2	2.6	0.5	0
Cloves, ground	1 tsp	7	0.4	0.1	1.3	0.7
Cocktail mix, non-alcoholic	1 fl oz	103	0	0.1	25.8	0
Cocoa mix, powder	1 serving	113	1.1	1.7	24	1
Cocoa mix, powder, unsweetened	1 tbsp	12	0.7	1.1	2.9	1.8
Coconut meat	1 cup, shredded	283	26.8	2.7	12.2	7.2
Coconut milk	1 cup	552	57.2	5.5	13.3	5.3
Coffee, brewed, decaf	1 cup	0	0	0.2	0	0
Coffee, brewed, regular	1 cup	2	0	0.3	0	0
Coffee, café au lait	8 fl oz.	65	2.5	1	6	0
Coffee, cappuccino	8 fl oz.	70	4	1	6	0
Coffee, espresso	1 shot	4	0	0	1	0
Coffee, instant, decaf	1 tsp	0	0	0	0	0
Coffee, instant, regular	1 tsp, dry	2	0	0.1	0.4	0

NUTRITIONAL INFORMATION

Nutrition values for fat, protein, carbohydrates, and fiber are listed in grams per serving.
Serving sizes and values are approximate.

FOOD ITEM	Serving Size	Cal.	Fat	Protein	Carbs	Fiber

C (cont.)

FOOD ITEM	Serving Size	Cal.	Fat	Protein	Carbs	Fiber
Coffee, latte	8 fl oz.	100	5	0	8	0
Coffee, mocha	8 fl oz.	180	12	1	16	0
Coffeecake	2.5 oz.	230	7	3.8	38	3.8
Coleslaw	1/2 cup	41	1.6	0.8	7.4	0.9
Collards	1 cup, chopped	11	0.2	0.9	2	1.3
Conch, baked or broiled	1 cup, sliced	165	1.5	33.4	2.2	0
Cookies, animal crackers	1 cookie	22	0.7	0.3	3.6	0.1
Cookies, brownies	3.5 oz.	430	25	1	52	1.2
Cookies, butter	1 cookie	23	0.9	0.3	3.4	0
Cookies, chocolate chip, deli fresh baked	1 cookie	275	15	0	37.5	1
Cookies, chocolate chip, commercial	1 cookie	130	6.9	0.9	16.7	0.9
Cookies, chocolate chip, refrigerated dough	1 portion	128	5.9	1.3	17.8	0.4
Cookies, chocolate wafers	1 wafer	26	0.8	0.4	4.3	0.2
Cookies, fig bars	1 cookie	150	3.1	1.6	30.5	2
Cookies, fudge	1 cookie	73	0.8	1.1	16.4	0.6
Cookies, gingersnap	1 cookie	29	0.7	0.4	5.4	0.2
Cookies, graham, plain or honey	2 1/2" square	30	0.7	0.5	5.3	0.2
Cookies, marshmallow w/ chocolate coating	1 cookie	118	4.7	1.1	19	0.6
Cookies, molasses	1 cookie	138	4.1	1.8	23.6	0.3
Cookies, oatmeal	1 cookie	238	8.8	2.5	37.5	2
Cookies, oatmeal w/ raisins	1 cookie	238	8.8	2.5	37.5	2
Cookies, oatmeal, commercial, iced	1 cookie	123	4.8	1.4	18.4	0.6
Cookies, oatmeal, refrigerated dough	1 portion	68	3	0.9	9.5	0.4
Cookies, peanut butter sandwich	1 cookie	67	3	1.2	9.2	0.3
Cookies, peanut butter, refrigerated dough	1 portion	73	4	1.3	8.3	0.2
Cookies, sugar	1 cookie	66	3.3	0.8	8.4	0.2
Cookies, sugar wafers w/ cream filling	1 wafer	46	2.2	0.4	6.3	0.1
Cookies, sugar, refrigerated dough	1 portion	113	5.4	1.1	15.3	0.2
Cookies, vanilla wafers	1 wafer	28	1.2	0.3	4.3	0.1
Coriander leaves	9 sprigs	5	0.1	0.4	0.7	0.6
Corn flour, yellow	1 cup	416	4.3	10.6	86.9	0
Corn, sweet, white	1 ear	77	1.1	2.9	17.1	2.4
Corn, sweet, yellow	1 ear	77	1.1	2.9	17.1	2.4
Corn, sweet, white, cream style	1 cup	184	1	4.5	46.4	3.1
Corn, sweet, yellow, cream style	1 cup	184	1	4.5	46.4	3.1
Cornnuts	1 oz	126	4.4	2.4	20.4	2
Cornstarch	1 cup	488	0.1	0.3	116.8	1.2
Couscous, cooked	1 cup	176	0.2	6	36.5	0.1
Cowpeas (blackeyes), cooked	1 cup	160	0.6	5.2	33.5	8.2
Cowpeas, cat jang, cooked	1 cup	200	1.2	14	34.7	6.2
Cowpeas, leafy tips	1 cup, chopped	10	0.1	1.5	1.7	0
Crab, Alaska king, raw	1 leg	144	1	31.5	0	0
Crab, blue, canned	1 cup	134	1.6	27.7	0	0
Crab, dungeness, cooked	1 crab	140	1.6	28.4	1.2	0
Crabapples	1 cup, sliced	84	0.3	0.4	21.9	0
Crackers w/ cheese filling	6 crackers	191	9.5	3.5	22.9	0.7
Crackers w/ peanut butter filling	6 cracker	193	9.8	4.8	22.1	1.3
Crackers, cheese, regular	6 crackers	312	15.7	6.3	36.1	1.5
Crackers, graham	1 cracker	30	0.5	6	5	2
Crackers, matzo, plain	1 matzo	112	0.4	2.8	23.7	0.9

Nutrition values for fat, protein, carbohydrates, and fiber are listed in grams per serving.
Serving sizes and values are approximate.

FOOD ITEM	Serving Size	Cal.	Fat	Protein	Carbs	Fiber
C (cont.)						
Crackers, matzo, whole-wheat	1 matzo	100	0.4	3.7	22.4	3.3
Crackers, melba toast	1 cup	129	1.1	4	25.3	2.1
Crackers, milk	1 cracker	50	1.7	0.8	7.7	0.2
Crackers, regular	1 cup, bite size	311	15.7	4.6	37.8	1
Crackers, rusk toast	1 rusk	41	0.7	1.4	7.2	0
Crackers, rye	1 cracker	37	0.1	1.1	8.8	2.5
Crackers, saltines	1 cracker	20	0.1	0.5	4.1	0.1
Crackers, soda	1 cracker	60	2	6	10	2
Crackers, wheat	1 cracker	9	0.4	0.1	1.3	0.1
Crackers, wheat, sandwich w/ peanut butter	1 cracker	35	1.8	0.9	3.7	0.3
Crackers, whole-wheat	1 cracker	18	0.7	0.3	2.7	0.4
Cranberries	1 cup, whole	44	0.1	0.4	11.6	4.4
Cranberry juice cocktail	1 cup	144	0.3	0	36.4	0.3
Cranberry-apple juice	1 cup	174	0.1	0.2	44.3	0.2
Cranberry-grape juice	1 cup	137	0.2	0.5	34.3	0.2
Crayfish, wild, raw	8 crayfish	21	0.3	4.3	0	0
Cream cheese	1 tbsp	51	5.1	1.1	0.4	0
Cream of tartar	1 tsp	8	0	0	1.8	0
Cream, half & half	1 tbsp	20	1.7	0.4	0.6	0
Cream, heavy whipping	1 cup, fluid	821	88.1	4.9	6.6	0
Crepes	1 crepe	120	6	2	14	1
Croissants, apple	1 croissant	145	5	4.2	21.1	1.4
Croissants, butter	1 croissant	115	6	2.3	13	0.7
Croissants, cheese	1 croissant	174	8.8	3.9	19.7	1.1
Croutons, plain	1 cup	122	2	3.6	22.1	1.5
Croutons, seasoned	1 cup	186	7.3	4.3	25.4	2
Cucumber	1 cucumber	45	0.3	2	10.9	1.5
Cucumber, peeled	1 cup, sliced	14	0.2	0.7	2.6	0.8
Cumin seed	1 tsp	8	0.5	0.4	0.9	0.2
Currants, black	1 cup	71	0.5	1.6	17.2	0
Currants, red & white	1 cup	63	0.2	1.6	15.5	4.8
Curry powder	1 tsp	7	0.3	0.3	1.2	0.7
D						
Dandelion greens	1 cup, chopped	25	0.4	1.5	5.1	1.9
Danish pastry, cheese, 4 1/4" diameter	1 pastry	266	15.5	5.7	26.4	0.7
Danish pastry, cinnamon, 4 1/4" diameter	1 pastry	262	14.5	4.5	29	0.8
Danish pastry, fruit, 4 1/4" diameter	1 pastry	263	13	3.8	33.9	1.3
Danish pastry, nut, 4 1/4" diameter	1 pastry	280	16.4	4.6	29.7	1.3
Danish pastry, raspberry, 4 1/4" diameter	1 pastry	263	13.1	3.8	33.9	1.3
Deer, ground, raw	1 oz	45	2	6.2	0	0
Deer, raw	1 oz	34	0.7	6.5	0	0
Doughnuts, chocolate coated or frosted	1 doughnut	133	8.7	1.4	13.4	0.6
Doughnuts, chocolate, sugared or glazed	1 doughnut	250	11.9	2.7	34.4	1.3
Doughnuts, french crullers	1 cruller	169	7.5	1.3	24.4	0.5
Doughnuts, plain	1 doughnut, stick	219	11.9	2.6	25.8	0.8
Doughnuts, wheat, sugared or glazed	1 doughnut	101	5.4	1.8	11.9	0.6
Duck liver, raw	1 liver	60	2	8.2	1.6	0
Duck, meat only, roasted	1/2 duck	444	24.7	51.9	0	0
Duck, white pekin, breast w/skin. roasted	1/2 breast	242	13	29.4	0	0

NUTRITIONAL INFORMATION

Nutrition values for fat, protein, carbohydrates, and fiber are listed in grams per serving.
Serving sizes and values are approximate.

FOOD ITEM	Serving Size	Cal.	Fat	Protein	Carbs	Fiber
D (cont.)						
Duck, skinless, raw	1/2 duck	400	18	55.4	0	0
Durian	1 cup, chopped	357	13	3.6	65.8	9.2
E						
Eclairs w/ chocolate glaze	1 éclair	293	17.6	7.2	27.1	0.7
Eel, mixed species, raw	3 oz	156	9.9	15.7	0	0
Egg noodles, cooked	1 cup	213	2.3	7.6	39.7	1.8
Egg substitute, liquid	1 tbsp	13	0.5	1.9	0.1	0
Egg white, fried	1 large	92	7	6.3	0.4	0
Egg white, raw	1 large	17	0.1	3.6	0.2	0
Egg yolk, raw	1 large	53	4.4	2.6	0.6	0
Egg, hard-boiled	1 cup, chopped	211	14.4	17.1	1.5	0
Egg, omelette	1 large	93	7.3	6.5	0.4	0
Egg, poached	1 large	74	4.9	6.3	0.4	0
Egg, raw	1 large	85	5.8	7.3	0.4	0
Egg, scrambled	1 cup	365	26.9	24.4	4.8	0
Eggnog	8 fl oz	343	19	9.6	34	0
Eggplant	1 eggplant	110	0.9	4.6	26.1	15.6
Elderberries	1 cup	106	0.7	1	26.7	10.2
Elk, ground, raw	1 oz	49	2.5	6.2	0	0
Elk, raw	1 oz	31	0.4	6.5	0	0
Endive	1 head	87	1	6.4	17.2	15.9
English muffins, plain	1 muffin	134	1	4.4	26.2	1.5
English muffins, cinnamon-raisin	1 muffin	139	1.5	4.2	48.7	1.7
English muffins, wheat	1 muffin	127	1.1	5	25.5	2.6
English muffins, whole-wheat	1 muffin	134	1.4	5.8	26.6	4.4
English muffins, whole-wheat/multi-grain	1 muffin	155	1.2	6	30.5	1.8
European chestnuts, peeled	1 oz	56	0.4	0.5	12.5	0
European chestnuts, unpeeled	1 oz	60	0.6	0.7	12.9	2.3
F						
Farina, cooked	1 cup	471	0.1	3.3	24.4	0.7
Fast Food, biscuit w/ egg	1 biscuit	373	22.1	11.6	31.9	0.8
Fast Food, biscuit w/ egg & bacon	1 biscuit	458	31.1	17	28.6	0.8
Fast Food, biscuit w/ egg, bacon & cheese	1 biscuit	477	31.4	16.3	33.4	0.1
Fast Food, biscuit w/ sausage	1 biscuit	485	31.8	12.1	40	1.4
Fast Food, caramel sundae	1 sundae	304	9.3	7.3	49.3	0
Fast Food, cheeseburger, large, double patty	1 sandwich	704	43.7	38	39.7	1
Fast Food, cheeseburger, large, single patty	1 sandwich	563	32.9	28.2	38.4	1
Fast Food, corndog	1 corndog	460	18.9	16.8	55.8	1
Fast Food, croissant w/ egg, cheese	1 croissant	368	24.7	12.8	24.3	1
Fast Food, croissant w/ egg, cheese, bacon	1 croissant	413	28.4	16.2	23.6	1
Fast Food, croissant w/ egg, cheese, sausage	1 croissant	523	38.2	20.3	24.7	1
Fast Food, Danish pastry, cheese	1 pastry	353	24.6	5.8	28.7	1.5
Fast Food, Danish pastry, cinnamon	1 pastry	349	16.7	4.8	46.9	1.5
Fast Food, Danish pastry, fruit	1 pastry	335	15.9	4.8	45.1	1.5
Fast Food, fish sandwich w/ tartar sauce	1 sandwich	431	22.8	16.9	41	1
Fast Food, french toast sticks	5 pieces	513	29	8.3	57.9	2.7
Fast Food, fried chicken, boneless	6 pieces	285	18.1	15	15.7	0.9
Fast Food, hamburger, large, double patty	1 sandwich	540	26.6	34.3	40.3	2.1

Nutrition values for fat, protein, carbohydrates, and fiber are listed in grams per serving.
Serving sizes and values are approximate.

FOOD ITEM	Serving Size	Cal.	Fat	Protein	Carbs	Fiber
F (cont.)						
Fast Food, hamburger, large, single patty	1 sandwich	425	20.9	23	36.7	2.1
Fast Food, hot fudge sundae	1 sundae	284	8.6	5.6	47.7	0
Fast Food, hot dog w/ chili	1 hot dog	296	13.4	13.5	31.3	1
Fast Food, hot dog, plain	1 hot dog	242	14.5	10.4	18	1
Fast Food, McDonald's Big Mac® w/ cheese	1 serving	560	30	25	46	3.1
Fast Food, McDonald's Big Mac® w/o cheese	1 serving	495	25.4	23.2	43.3	2.7
Fast Food, McDonald's cheeseburger	1 serving	310	12	15	35	1
Fast Food, McDonald's Chicken McGrill®	1 serving	400	16	27	38	3
Fast Food, McDonald's Crispy Chicken	1 serving	500	23	24	50	3
Fast Food, McDonald's Filet-o-Fish®	1 serving	400	18	14	42	1
Fast Food, McDonald's french fries	1 medium	350	11	4	47	5
Fast Food, McDonald's hamburger	1 serving	260	9	13	33	1
Fast Food, McDonald's 1/4 Pounder®,cheese	1 serving	510	25	29	43	3
Fast Food, McDonald's 1/4 Pounder®	1 serving	420	18	24	40	3
Fast Food, onion rings, 8-9 rings	1 portion	276	15.5	3.7	31.3	3.3
Fast Food, strawberry sundae	1 sundae	268	7.8	6.3	44.6	0
Fast Food, submarine sandwich w/ cold cuts	1 submarine 6"	456	18.6	21.8	51	4
Fast Food, submarine sandwich w/ roast beef	1 submarine 6"	410	13	28.6	44.3	4
Fast Food, submarine sandwich w/ tuna	1 submarine 6"	584	28	29.7	55.4	4
Fast Food, vanilla soft-serve w/ cone	1 cone	164	6.1	3.9	24.1	0.1
Fennel bulb	1 cup, sliced	27	0.2	1.1	6.3	2.7
Fennel seed	1 tbsp	20	0.9	0.9	3	2.3
Fenugreek seed	1 tbsp	36	0.7	2.6	6.5	2.7
Figs	1 medium	37	0.2	0.4	9.6	1.5
Figs, dried	1 fig	21	0.01	0.3	5.3	0.8
Fireweed leaves	1 cup, chopped	24	0.6	1.1	4.4	2.4
Fish oil, cod liver	1 tbsp	123	13.6	0	0	0
Fish oil, herring	1 tbsp	123	13.6	0	0	0
Fish oil, menhaden	1 tbsp	123	13.6	0	0	0
Fish oil, salmon	1 tbsp	123	13.6	0	0	0
Fish oil, sardine	1 tbsp	123	13.6	0	0	0
Fish, bluefin tuna, raw	3 oz	122	4.2	19.8	0	0
Fish, bluefish, raw	3 oz	105	3.6	17	0	0
Fish, butterfish, raw	3 oz	124	6.8	14.7	0	0
Fish, carp, raw	3 oz	108	4.8	15.2	0	0
Fish, catfish, raw	3 oz	81	2.4	13.9	0	0
Fish, cod, atlantic, raw	3 oz	70	0.6	15.1	0	0
Fish, croaker, atlantic, raw	3 oz	88	2.7	15.1	0	0
Fish, flatfish, raw	3 oz	77	1	16	0	0
Fish, gefilte fish	1 piece	35	0.7	3.8	3.1	0
Fish, grouper, mixed species, raw	3 oz	78	0.9	16.5	0	0
Fish, haddock, raw	3 oz	74	0.6	16.1	0	0
Fish, halibut, raw	3 oz	94	1.9	17.7	0	0
Fish, herring, atlantic, raw	3 oz	134	7.7	15.3	0	0
Fish, herring, pacific, raw	3 oz	166	11.8	13.9	0	0
Fish, mackerel, atlantic, raw	3 oz	174	11.8	15.8	0	0
Fish, mackerel, king, raw	3 oz	89	1.7	17.2	0	0
Fish, mackerel, pacific, raw	3 oz	134	6.7	17.1	0	0
Fish, mackerel, spanish, raw	3 oz	118	5.4	16.4	0	1
Fish, milkfish, raw	3 oz	126	5.7	17.5	0	0

NUTRITIONAL INFORMATION

Nutrition values for fat, protein, carbohydrates, and fiber are listed in grams per serving.
Serving sizes and values are approximate.

FOOD ITEM	Serving Size	Cal.	Fat	Protein	Carbs	Fiber
F (cont.)						
Fish, monkfish, raw	3 oz	65	1.3	12.3	0	0
Fish, ocean perch, atlantic, raw	3 oz	80	1.4	15.8	0	0
Fish, perch, mixed species, raw	3 oz	77	0.8	16.5	0	0
Fish, pike, northern, raw	3 oz	75	0.6	16.4	0	0
Fish, pollock, atlantic, raw	3 oz	78	0.8	16.5	0	0
Fish, pout, ocean, raw	3 oz	67	0.8	14.1	0	0
Fish, rainbow smelt, raw	3 oz	82	2.1	15	0	0
Fish, rockfish, pacific, raw	3 oz	80	1.3	15.9	0	0
Fish, roe, mixed species, raw	1 tbsp	20	0.9	3.1	0.2	0
Fish, sablefish, raw	3 oz	166	13	11.4	0	0
Fish, salmon, atlantic, farmed, raw	3 oz	156	9.2	16.9	0	0
Fish, salmon, atlantic, wild, raw	3 oz	121	5.4	16.9	0	0
Fish, salmon, chinook, raw	3 oz	152	8.9	16.9	0	0
Fish, salmon, pink, raw	3 oz	99	2.9	16.9	0	0
Fish, sea bass, mixed species, raw	3 oz	82	1.7	15.7	0	0
Fish, seatrout, mixed species, raw	3 oz	88	3.1	14.2	0	0
Fish, shad, raw	3 oz	167	11.7	14.4	0	0
Fish, skipjack tuna, raw	3 oz	88	0.9	18.7	0	0
Fish, snapper, mixed species, raw	3 oz	85	1.1	17.4	0	0
Fish, striped bass, raw	3 oz	82	2	15.1	0	0
Fish, striped mullet	3 oz	99	3.2	16.4	0	0
Fish, sturgeon, mixed species, raw	3 oz	89	3.4	13.7	0	0
Fish, swordfish, raw	3 oz	103	3.4	16.8	0	0
Fish, trout, mixed species, raw	3 oz	126	5.6	17.7	0	0
Fish, white sucker, raw	3 oz	78	2	14.2	0	0
Fish, whitefish, raw	3 oz	114	5	16.2	0	0
Fish, wolffish, atlantic, raw	3 oz	82	2	14.9	0	0
Fish, yellowfin tuna, raw	3 oz	93	0.9	19.8	0	0
Fish, yellowtail, mixed species, raw	3 oz	124	4.5	19.7	0	0
Flan, caramel custard	5 1/2 oz.	303	12	4	43	0
Flaxseed	1 tbsp	59	4.1	2.3	4.1	3.3
Flaxseed oil	1 tbsp	120	13.6	0	0	0
Frankfurter	1 serving	151	13.4	5.3	2.2	0
Frankfurter, beef	1 frankfurter	188	16.9	6.4	2.3	0
Frankfurter, beef & pork	1 frankfurter	174	15.8	6.6	1	1.4
Frankfurter, chicken	1 frankfurter	116	8.8	5.8	3.1	0
Frankfurter, meat	1 frankfurter	151	13.4	5.3	2.2	0
Frankfurter, meatless	1 frankfurter	163	9.6	13.7	5.4	2.7
Frankfurter, pork	1 frankfurter	204	18	9.7	0.2	0.1
Frankfurter, turkey	1 frankfurter	102	8	6.4	0.7	0
French fries, frozen, unprepared, 18 fries	1 serving	170	6.7	2.8	27.7	3.4
French toast , frozen, ready-to-heat	1 piece	126	3.6	4.3	18.9	0.6
Frosting, creamy chocolate	2 tbsp	164	7.3	0.5	26.1	0.4
Frosting, creamy vanilla	2 tbsp	160	6.3	0	25.6	0
Frozen yogurt, chocolate, soft-serve	1/2 cup	115	4.3	2.9	17.9	1.6
Frozen yogurt, vanilla, soft-serve	1/2 cup	117	4	2.9	17.4	0
Fruit cocktail, canned	1 cup	229	0.2	1	59.5	2.9
Fruit punch, prepared from concentrate	8 fl oz.	124	0.5	0.2	30.2	0.2
Fruit salad, canned in syrup	1 cup	186	0.2	0.9	48.7	2.6
Fruit salad, canned in water	1 cup	74	0.2	0.9	19.3	2.5

NUTRITIONAL INFORMATION

Nutrition values for fat, protein, carbohydrates, and fiber are listed in grams per serving.
Serving sizes and values are approximate.

FOOD ITEM	Serving Size	Cal.	Fat	Protein	Carbs	Fiber
G						
Garden cress, raw	1 cup	16	0.3	1.3	2.7	0.6
Garlic	1 clove	4	0	0.2	1	0.1
Garlic powder	1 tsp	9	0	0.5	2	0.3
Gelatin dessert mix, prepared w/ water	1/2 cup	84	0	1.6	19.1	0
Gin, 80 Proof	1 fl oz.	73	0	0	0	0
Ginger root	1 tsp	2	0	0	0.4	0
Ginger, ground	1 tsp	6	0.1	0.2	1.3	0.2
Ginkgo nuts	1 oz	52	0.5	1.2	10.7	0
Ginkgo nuts, dried	1 oz	99	0.6	2.9	20.5	0
Goose liver, raw	1 liver	125	4	15.4	5.9	0
Goose, meat & skin, roasted	1 cup chopped	427	30.7	35.2	0	0
Goose, meat only, roasted	1 cup chopped	340	18.1	41.4	0	0
Gourd, white-flowered	1 gourd	108	0.2	4.8	26.1	0
Granola bars, hard, plain	1 bar	134	5.6	2.9	18.3	1.5
Granola bars, soft, plain	1 bar	126	4.9	2.1	19.1	1.3
Grape juice	8 fl oz.	160	0	0	40	0
Grapefruit	1/2 fruit	50	0	1	12	3
Grapefruit juice, sweetened	8 fl oz.	125	0	0	32.6	0
Grapefruit juice, unsweetened	8 fl oz.	91	0.2	1.2	21.5	0
Grapes, canned, heavy syrup	1 cup	187	0.3	1.2	50.3	1.5
Grapes, red or green	1 cup	106	0.2	1.1	27.9	1.4
Gravy mushroom, canned	1 can	149	8.1	3.8	16.3	1.2
Gravy, au jus, canned	1 can	48	0.6	3.6	7.5	0
Gravy, beef, canned	1 can	154	6.9	10.9	14	1.2
Gravy, chicken, canned	1 can	235	17	5.8	16.2	1.2
Gravy, turkey, canned	1 can	152	6.2	7.7	15.2	1.2
Guacamole dip	2 tbsp	50	4	12	4	0
Guavas	1 fruit	37	0.5	1.4	7.8	3
H						
Ham, chopped	1 slice	50	2.9	4.6	1.2	0
Ham, minced	1 slice	55	4.3	3.4	0.4	0
Ham, sliced	1 slice	46	2.4	4.6	1.1	0.4
Hazlenuts, dry roasted	1 oz	183	17.7	4.2	5	2.7
Hazlenuts, blanched	1 oz	178	17.3	3.9	4.8	3.1
Hominy, canned, white	1 cup	119	1.5	2.4	23.5	4.1
Hominy, canned, yellow	1 cup	115	1.4	2.4	22.8	4
Honey	1 tbsp	64	0	0.1	17.3	0
Honeydew melons	1 cup, diced	61	0.2	0.9	15.5	1.4
Horseradish	1 tsp	2	0	0.1	0.6	0.2
Hot chocolate	8 fl oz.	200	10	9	25	3
Hummus	1 tbsp	23	1.3	1.1	2	0.8
Hush puppies	1 hush puppy	74	2.9	1.7	10.1	0.6
I						
Ice cream cone, rolled or sugar type	1 cone	40	0.4	0.8	8.4	0.2
Ice cream cone, wafer or cake type	1 cone	17	0.3	0.3	3.2	0.1
Ice cream, chocolate	1/2 cup	143	7.3	2.5	18.6	0.8
Ice cream, strawberry	1/2 cup	127	5.5	2.1	18.2	0.6
Ice cream, vanilla	1/2 cup	144	7.9	2.5	16.9	0.5

NUTRITIONAL INFORMATION

Nutrition values for fat, protein, carbohydrates, and fiber are listed in grams per serving.
Serving sizes and values are approximate.

FOOD ITEM	Serving Size	Cal.	Fat	Protein	Carbs	Fiber
I (cont.)						
Iced tea, pre-sweetened	8 fl oz.	100	0	0	25	0
Iced tea, unsweetened	8 fl oz.	2	0	0	0	0
Italian seasoning	1 tsp	4	0	0	1	0
J						
Jams and preserves	1 tbsp	56	0	0.1	13.8	0.2
Japanese chestnuts	1 oz	44	0.2	0.6	9.9	0
Japanese soba noodles, cooked	1 cup	113	0.1	5.7	24.4	1.7
Japanese ramen noodles, packaged, dry	1 serving	195	7.3	4	28	1
Jellies	1 tbsp	55	0	0	14.4	0.2
K						
Kale	1 cup, chopped	34	0.5	2.2	6.7	1.3
Kiwifruit	1 medium	45	0	2	11	5
Kumquats	1 fruit	13	0.2	0.4	3	1.2
L						
Lamb, cubed, raw	1 oz	38	1.5	5.7	0	0
Lamb, foreshank, raw	1 oz	57	3.8	5.4	0	0
Lamb, ground, raw	1 oz	80	6.6	4.7	0	0
Lamb, leg, shank half, raw	1 oz	52	3.3	5.4	0	0
Lamb, leg, sirloin half, raw	1 oz	74	5.9	4.9	0	0
Lamb, leg, whole, choice, raw	1 oz	65	4.8	5.1	0	0
Lamb, loin, choice, raw	1 oz	79	6.4	4.9	0	0
Lamb, rib, choice, raw	1 oz	97	8.7	4.3	0	0
Lamb, shoulder, arm, raw	1 oz	69	5.4	4.9	0	0
Lamb, shoulder, blade, raw	1 oz	69	5.4	4.8	0	0
Lamb, shoulder, whole, raw	1 oz	69	5.4	4.8	0	0
Lard	1 tbsp	115	12.8	0	0	0
Leeks	1 leek	54	0.3	1.3	12.6	1.6
Lemon juice	1 cup	61	0	0.9	21.1	1
Lemon juice, canned or bottled	1 tbsp	3	0	0.1	1	0.1
Lemon pepper seasoning	1 tsp	7	0	0	1	0
Lemonade powder	1 scoop	102	0	0	26.9	0
Lemonade, pink concentrate, prepared	8 fl oz.	99	0	0.2	25.9	0
Lemonade, white concentrate, prepared	8 fl oz.	131	0.1	0.2	34	0.2
Lemons w/ peel	1 fruit	22	0.3	1.3	11.6	5.1
Lentils, cooked	1 cup	230	0.7	17.8	39.8	15.6
Lentils, sprouted, raw	1 cup	82	0.4	6.9	17	0
Lettuce, green leaf	1 cup, shredded	5	0.1	0.5	1	0.5
Lettuce, iceberg	1 cup, shredded	10	0.1	0.7	2.2	0.9
Lettuce, red leaf	1 cup, shredded	3	0	0.2	0.4	0.2
Lettuce, romaine	1 cup, shredded	8	0.1	0.6	1.5	1
Lime juice	1 cup	62	0.2	1	20.7	1
Limes	1 fruit	20	0.1	0.5	7.1	1.9
Liverwurst, pork	1 slice	59	5.1	2.5	0.4	0
Lobster, northern, raw	1 lobster	135	1.3	28.2	0.8	0
Luncheon meat, beef, loaved	1 oz.	87	7.4	4.1	0.8	0
Luncheon meat, beef, thin sliced	1 oz.	50	1.1	8	1.6	0
Luncheon meat, meatless slices	1 slice	26	1.6	2.5	0.6	0

Nutrition values for fat, protein, carbohydrates, and fiber are listed in grams per serving. Serving sizes and values are approximate.

FOOD ITEM	Serving Size	Cal.	Fat	Protein	Carbs	Fiber
L (cont.)						
Luncheon meat, pork & chicken, minced	1 oz	56	3.9	4.3	0.4	0
Luncheon meat, pork & ham, minced	1 oz	88	7.45	3.75	1.3	0
Luncheon meat, pork or beef	1 oz.	99	9	3.5	0.6	0
Luncheon meat, pork, canned	1 oz.	95	8.6	3.5	0.6	0
Luncheon meat, pork, ham & chicken, minced	1 oz	87	7.6	3.7	0.8	0
Luncheon sausage, pork & beef	1 oz.	74	5.9	4.3	0.4	0
M						
Macadamia nuts	1 oz. (10-12 nuts)	203	21.5	2.2	3.6	2.3
Macaroni and cheese, commercial, prepared	1 cup	259	2.6	11.3	47.5	1.5
Macaroni, cooked	1 cup	197	0.9	6.6	39.6	1.8
Malt drink mix, dry	3 heaping tsp	87	1.7	2.4	15.9	0.2
Malt beverage	8 fl oz.	144	0.2	0.7	32.2	0
Mangos	1 fruit	135	0.6	1.1	35.2	3.7
Maraschino cherries	1 cherry	8	0	0	2.1	0.2
Margarine, fat-free spread	1 tbsp	6	0.4	0	0.6	0
Margarine, stick	1 tbsp	100	11.2	0	0.3	0
Margarine, stick, unsalted	1 tbsp	102	11.4	0.1	0.1	0
Margarine, tub	1 tbsp	102	11.4	0.1	0.1	0
Martini	1 fl oz	69	0	0	0.6	0
Mayonnaise	1 tbsp	100	11	0	0	0
Milk, 1% low fat	1 cup	102	2.4	8.2	12.2	0
Milk, 2% low fat	1 cup	138	4.9	9.7	13.5	0
Milk, buttermilk, cultured, reduced fat	1 cup	137	4.9	10	13	0
Milk, chocolate	1 cup	208	8.5	7.9	25.9	2
Milk, dry, non fat, instant	1/3 cup dry	82	0.1	8	12	0
Milk, evaporated	1/2 cup	169	9.5	8.5	12.6	0
Milk, skim or nonfat	1 cup	83	0.2	8.3	12.2	0
Milk, canned, sweetened condensed	1 cup	982	26.6	24.2	166.5	0
Milk, whole	1 cup	146	7.9	7.9	11	0
Milkshake dry mix, vanilla	1 envelope packet	69	0.5	4.9	11.1	0.3
Millet	1 cup	756	8.4	22	145.7	17
Miso soup	1 cup	547	16.5	32.1	72.8	14.9
Mixed nuts	1 cup	814	70.5	23.7	34.7	12.3
Molasses	1 tablespoon	58	0	0	15	0
Muffins, apple bran	1 muffin	300	3	1	61	1
Muffins, banana nut	1 muffin	480	24	3	60	2
Muffins, blueberry	1 muffin	313	7.3	6.2	54.2	2.9
Muffins, chocolate chip	1 muffin	510	24	2	69	4
Muffins, corn	1 muffin	345	9.5	6.6	57.5	3.8
Muffins, oat-bran	1 muffin	305	8.3	7.9	54.5	5.2
Muffins, plain	1 muffin	242	9.1	3.8	36.3	1.5
Mushrooms	1 cup, pieces	15	0.2	2.2	2.3	0.8
Mushrooms, enoki	1 large	2	0	0.1	0.4	0.1
Mushrooms, oyster	1 large	55	0.8	6.1	9.2	3.6
Mushrooms, portobello	1 large	0	0	0	0	0
Mushrooms, shiitake	1 mushroom	11	0	0.3	2.7	0.4
Mussel, blue, raw	1 cup	129	3.4	17.8	5.5	0
Mustard greens	1 cup, chopped	15	0.1	1.5	2.7	1.8
Mustard seed, yellow	1 tbsp	53	3.2	2.8	3.9	1.6

Nutrition values for fat, protein, carbohydrates, and fiber are listed in grams per serving.
Serving sizes and values are approximate.

FOOD ITEM	Serving Size	Cal.	Fat	Protein	Carbs	Fiber
M (cont.)						
Mustard spinach	1 cup, chopped	33	0.5	3.3	5.9	4.2
Mustard, prepared, yellow	1 tsp	3	0.2	0.2	0.4	0.2
N						
Natto (fermented soybeans)	1 cup	371	19.3	31	25.1	9.5
Nectarines	1 fruit	60	0.4	1.4	14.3	2.3
New Zealand spinach	1 cup, chopped	8	0.1	0.8	1.4	0
Nutmeg, ground	1 tsp	12	0.8	0.1	1.1	0.5
O						
Oat bran	1 cup	231	6.6	16.3	62.2	14.5
Oatmeal, instant, prepared w/ water	1 cup	129	2.1	5.4	22.4	3.7
Oil, canola & corn	1 tbsp	124	14	0	0	0
Oil, canola & soybean	1 tbsp	120	13.6	0	0	0
Oil, coconut	1 tbsp	120	13.6	0	0	0
Oil, corn, peanut & olive	1 tbsp	120	13.6	0	0	0
Oil, olive	1 tbsp	119	13.5	0	0	0
Oil, peanut	1 tbsp	119	13.5	0	0	0
Oil, sesame	1 tbsp	120	13.6	0	0	0
Oil, soy	1 tbsp	120	13.6	0	0	0
Oil, vegetable, almond	1 tbsp	120	13.6	0	0	0
Oil, vegetable, cocoa butter	1 tbsp	120	13.6	0	0	0
Oil, vegetable, coconut	1 tbsp	117	13.6	0	0	0
Oil, vegetable, grapeseed	1 tbsp	120	13.6	0	0	0
Oil, vegetable, hazelnut	1 tbsp	120	13.6	0	0	0
Oil, vegetable, nutmeg butter	1 tbsp	120	13.6	0	0	0
Oil, vegetable, palm	1 tbsp	120	13.6	0	0	0
Oil, vegetable, poppyseed	1 tbsp	120	13.6	0	0	0
Oil, vegetable, rice bran	1 tbsp	120	13.6	0	0	0
Oil, vegetable, sheanut	1 tbsp	120	13.6	0	0	0
Oil, vegetable, tomatoseed	1 tbsp	120	13.6	0	0	0
Oil, vegetable, walnut	1 tbsp	1927	218	0	0	0
Okra	1 cup	31	0.1	2	7	3.2
Onion powder	1 tsp	8	0	0.2	1.9	0.1
Onions	1 cup, chopped	67	0.1	1.5	16.2	2.2
Onions, sweet	1 onion	106	0.3	2.7	25	3
Orange juice	8 fl oz	109	0.6	1.9	25	0.5
Orange marmalade	1 tbsp	49	0	0.1	13.3	0.1
Oranges	1 large	86	0.2	1.7	21.6	4.4
Oregano, dried	1 tsp, ground	6	0.2	0.2	1.2	0.8
Oyster, eastern, raw	3 oz.	50	1.3	4.4	4.6	0
Oyster, pacific, raw	3 oz.	69	1.9	8	4.2	0
P						
Pancakes, blueberry	1 pancake	84	3.5	2.3	11	0
Pancakes, buttermilk	1 pancake	86	3.5	2.6	10.9	0
Pancakes, plain, dry mix	1 pancake	74	1	2	13.9	0.5
Papayas	1 cup, cubed	55	0.2	0.9	13.7	2.5
Paprika	1 tsp	6	0.3	0.3	1.2	0.8
Parsley	1 cup	22	0.5	1.8	3.8	2

Nutrition values for fat, protein, carbohydrates, and fiber are listed in grams per serving.
Serving sizes and values are approximate.

FOOD ITEM	Serving Size	Cal.	Fat	Protein	Carbs	Fiber
P (cont.)						
Parsley, dried	1 tsp	1	0	0.1	0.2	0.1
Parsnips	1 cup, sliced	100	0.4	1.6	23.9	6.5
Passion-fruit	1 fruit	17	0.1	0.4	4.2	1.9
Pasta, corn, cooked	1 cup	176	1	3.6	39	6.7
Pasta, plain, cooked	1 cup	197	0.9	6.6	39.6	2.4
Pasta, spinach, cooked	1 cup	195	1.4	7.6	37.5	2.4
Pastrami, turkey	1 oz	40	1.8	5.2	0.5	0
Pate de foie gras	1 tbsp	60	5.7	1.5	0.6	0
Pate, chicken liver, canned	1 tbsp	26	1.7	1.7	0.9	0
Pate, goose liver, canned	1 tbsp	60	5.7	1.5	0.6	0
Peaches	1 large	61	0.4	1.4	15	2.4
Peaches, canned	1 cup, halved	59	0.1	1.1	14.9	3.2
Peanut butter, chunky	2 tbsp	188	16	7.7	6.9	2.6
Peanut butter, smooth	2 tbsp	188	16.1	8	6.3	1.9
Peanuts, dry roasted w/ salt	1 oz	166	14	6.7	6.1	2.3
Peanuts, raw	1 oz	161	13.9	7.3	4.5	2.4
Pears	1 pear	121	0.3	0.8	32.3	6.5
Pears, asian	1 pear	116	0.6	1.4	29.3	9.9
Pears, canned	1 cup	71	0.1	0.5	19.1	3.9
Peas, green, fresh, cooked	1 cup	134	0.3	8.5	25	8.8
Peas, green, frozen, cooked	1 cup	125	0.4	8.2	22.8	8.8
Peas, split, cooked	1 cup	231	0.7	16.3	41.3	16.3
Pecans	1 oz. (20 halves)	196	20.4	2.6	3.9	2.7
Pepper, black	1 tsp	5	0.1	0.2	1.4	0.6
Pepper, red or cayenne	1 tsp	6	0.3	0.2	1	0.5
Pepperoni	15 slices	135	11.7	5.9	1.2	0.4
Peppers, chili, green	1 cup	29	0.4	1	6.4	2.4
Peppers, chili, red	1 pepper	18	0.2	0.8	4	0.7
Peppers, chili, sun-dried	1 pepper	2	0	0.1	0.4	0.2
Peppers, jalapeno	1 pepper	4	0.1	0.2	0.8	0.4
Peppers, sweet, green	1 medium	24	0.2	1	5.5	2
Peppers, sweet, red	1 medium	31	0.3	1.1	7.2	2.4
Peppers, sweet, yellow	1 medium	32	0.2	1.2	7.5	1.1
Persimmons	1 fruit	32	0.1	0.2	8.4	0
Pheasant, boneless, raw	1/2 pheasant	724	37.2	90.8	0	0
Pheasant, breast, skinless, boneless, raw	1/2 breast	242	5.9	44.4	0	0
Pheasant, leg, skinless, boneless, raw	1 leg	143	4.6	23.8	0	0
Pheasant, skinless, raw	1/2 pheasant	468	12.8	83	0	0
Pickle relish, sweet	1 tbsp	20	0.1	0.1	5.3	0.2
Pickle, cucumber, sour	1 large 4"	15	0.3	0.4	3.1	1.6
Pickle, cucumber, sweet	1 large 4"	158	0.3	0.5	42.9	1.5
Pickles, cucumber, dill	1 large 4"	24	0.2	0.8	5.5	1.6
Pie crust, graham-cracker, baked	1 pie crust	1037	52.3	8.8	136.9	3.2
Pie, apple	1 piece	411	19.4	3.7	57.5	0
Pie, blueberry	1 piece	290	12.5	2.2	43.6	1.3
Pie, cherry	1 piece	325	13.8	2.5	49.7	1
Pie, lemon meringue	1 piece	303	9.8	1.7	53.3	1.4
Pie, pecan	1 piece	452	20.9	4.5	64.6	4
Pie, pumpkin	1 piece	229	10.4	4.3	29.8	2.9
Pine nuts	1 oz. (167 kernels)	191	19.3	3.8	3.7	1

Nutrition values for fat, protein, carbohydrates, and fiber are listed in grams per serving.
Serving sizes and values are approximate.

P (cont.)

FOOD ITEM	Serving Size	Cal.	Fat	Protein	Carbs	Fiber
Pineapple	1 fruit	227	0.6	2.5	59.6	6.6
Pineapple, canned	1 slice	15	0	0.2	3.9	0.4
Pita bread, whole wheat	1 pita	170	1.7	6.4	35.2	4.8
Pistachio nuts	1 oz (49 kernels)	161	13	6	7.6	2.9
Pizza, cheese	1 slice (3.7 oz.)	250	10	11	29	2
Pizza, pepperoni	1 slice (3.7 oz.)	288	15.2	11.7	26.1	1.7
Plantains	1 medium	218	0.7	2.3	57.1	4.1
Plums	1 fruit	30	0.2	0.5	7.5	0.9
Plums, canned	1 plum	19	0	0.2	5.1	0.4
Polenta	1/2 cup	220	2	2	24	1
Pomegranates	1 fruit	105	0.5	1.5	26.4	0.9
Popcorn cakes	1 cake	38	0.3	1	8	0.3
Popcorn, air-popped	1 cup	31	0.3	1	6.2	1.2
Popcorn, caramel-coated	1 oz	122	3.6	1.1	22.4	1.5
Popcorn, cheese	1 cup	58	3.7	1	5.7	1.1
Popcorn, oil-popped	1 cup	55	3.1	1	6.3	1.1
Popovers, dry mix	1 oz.	105	1.2	2.9	20	0.5
Poppy seed	1 tsp	15	1.3	0.5	0.7	0.3
Pork, cured, breakfast strips, cooked	3 slices	156	12.4	9.8	0.3	0
Pork, cured, ham, extra lean, canned	3 oz	116	4.1	17.9	0.4	0
Pork, cured, ham, patties	1 patty	205	18.4	8.3	1.1	0
Pork, cured, ham, extra lean, cooked	3 oz	140	6.5	18.6	0.4	0
Pork, cured, salt pork, raw	1 oz.	212	22.8	1.4	0	0
Pork, fresh ground, cooked	3 oz.	252	17.6	21.8	0	0
Pork, leg, rump half, cooked	3 oz.	214	12.1	24.5	0	0
Pork, leg, shank half, cooked	3 oz.	246	17	21.5	0	0
Pork, leg, whole, cooked	3 oz.	232	14.9	22.8	0	0
Pork, loin, blade, cooked	3 oz.	275	20.9	20.1	0	0
Pork, loin, center loin, cooked	3 oz.	199	11.4	22.3	0	0
Pork, loin, center rib, cooked	3 oz.	214	12.8	22.9	0	0
Pork, loin, sirloin, cooked	3 oz.	176	8	24.2	0	0
Pork, loin, tenderloin, cooked	3 oz.	147	5.1	23.6	0	0
Pork, loin, top loin, cooked	3 oz.	192	9.7	24.4	0	0
Pork, loin, whole, cooked	3 oz.	211	12.4	23	0	0
Pork, shoulder, arm, cooked	3 oz	238	18.1	17.3	0	0
Pork, shoulder, blade, cooked	3 oz	229	16	19.6	0	0
Pork, shoulder, whole, cooked	3 oz	248	18.2	19.8	0	0
Pork, spareribs, cooked	3 oz	337	25.7	24.7	0	0
Potato chips, barbecue	1 oz.	139	9.2	2.2	14.9	1.2
Potato chips, cheese	1 oz.	141	7.7	2.4	16.3	1.5
Potato chips, salted	1 oz.	152	9.8	1.9	15	1.3
Potato chips, sour cream & onion	1 oz.	151	9.6	2.3	14.6	1.5
Potato chips, reduced fat	1 oz.	134	5.9	2	18.9	1.7
Potato chips, unsalted	1 oz.	152	9.8	2	15	1.4
Potato flour	1 cup	571	0.5	11	132.9	9.4
Potato salad	1 cup	358	20.5	6.7	27.9	3.2
Potatoes	1 medium	164	0.2	4.3	37.2	4.7
Potatoes, baked, w/ skin	1 medium	160	0.2	4.3	36.5	3.8
Potatoes, baked, w/o skin	1 medium	143	0.2	2.8	33.3	3.3
Potatoes, mashed	1 cup	237	8.9	3.9	35.2	3.2

NUTRITIONAL INFORMATION

Nutrition values for fat, protein, carbohydrates, and fiber are listed in grams per serving.
Serving sizes and values are approximate.

FOOD ITEM	Serving Size	Cal.	Fat	Protein	Carbs	Fiber
P (cont.)						
Potatoes, red	1 medium	153	0.3	4	33.9	3.6
Potatoes, russet	1 medium	168	0.2	4.6	38.5	2.8
Potatoes, scalloped	1 cup	211	9	7	26.4	4.7
Potatoes, white	1 medium	149	0.2	3.6	33.5	5.1
Pretzels, hard, plain, salted	1 oz.	108	0.9	2.6	22.4	0.9
Prune juice	8 fl oz.	180	0	2	43	3
Pudding, banana	1/2 cup	154	2.5	4	29	0
Pudding, chocolate	1/2 cup	154	2.8	4.6	27.7	0
Pudding, coconut cream	1/2 cup	157	3.3	4.2	28.2	0.1
Pudding, lemon	1/2 cup	157	2.5	4	29.7	0
Pudding, rice	1/2 cup	163	2.4	4.8	30.6	0.1
Pudding, tapioca	1/2 cup	154	2.4	4.2	28.7	0
Pudding, vanilla	1/2 cup	148	2.5	4.3	27.2	0
Pumpkin	1 cup	30	0.1	1.2	7.5	0.6
Pumpkin pie mix	1 cup	281	0.4	2.9	71.3	22.4
Pumpkin, canned	1 cup	83	0.7	2.7	19.8	7.1
R						
Rabbit, cooked	3 oz	167	6.8	24.7	0	0
Radicchio	1 cup, shredded	9	0.1	0.6	1.8	0.4
Radishes	1 cup, sliced	19	0.1	0.8	3.9	1.9
Raisins	1 1/2 oz.	129	0.2	1.3	34	1.6
Raisins, golden	1 1/2 oz.	130	0.2	1.4	34.1	1.7
Raspberries	1 cup	64	0.8	1.5	14.7	8
Rhubarb	1 cup, diced	26	0.2	1.1	5.5	2.2
Rice cakes, brown rice, corn	1 cake	35	0.3	0.8	7.3	0.3
Rice cakes, brown rice, multi-grain	1 cake	35	0.3	0.8	7.2	0.3
Rice cakes, brown rice, plain	1 cake	35	0.3	0.7	7.3	0.4
Rice, brown, cooked	1 cup	218	1.6	4.5	45.8	3.5
Rice, white, cooked	1 cup	242	0.3	4.4	53.2	0.6
Rice, wild	1 cup	166	0.5	6.5	35	3
Rolls, dinner	1 roll	136	3.1	3.6	22.9	0.8
Rolls, dinner, wheat	1 roll	117	2.7	3.7	19.7	1.6
Rolls, dinner, whole-wheat	1 roll	114	2	3.7	21.9	3.2
Rolls, french	1 roll	119	1.8	3.7	21.5	0.1
Rolls, hamburger or hotdog	1 roll	120	1.9	4.1	21.3	0.9
Rolls, hard (incl. kaiser)	1 roll	126	1.8	4.2	22.6	1
Rolls, pumpernickel	1 roll	119	1.2	4.6	22.7	2.3
Rosemary	1 tsp	1	0	0	0.1	0.1
Rosemary, dried	1 tsp	4	0.2	0.1	0.8	0.5
Rum, 80 Proof	1 fl oz.	64	0	0	0	0
Rutabagas	1 cup, cubed	50	0.3	1.7	11.4	3.5
Rye	1 cup	566	4.2	24.9	117.9	24.7
Rye flour, dark	1 cup	415	3.4	18	88	28.9
Rye flour, light	1 cup	374	1.4	8.6	81.8	14.9
Rye flour, medium	1 cup	361	1.8	9.6	79	14.9
S						
Sage, ground	1 tsp	2	0.1	0.1	0.4	0.3
Sake	1 fl oz	39	0	0.1	1.5	0

Nutrition values for fat, protein, carbohydrates, and fiber are listed in grams per serving.
Serving sizes and values are approximate.

FOOD ITEM	Serving Size	Cal.	Fat	Protein	Carbs	Fiber
S (cont.)						
Salad dressing, 1000 island	1 tbsp	58	5.5	0.2	2.3	0.1
Salad dressing, bacon & tomato	1 tbsp	49	5.3	0.3	0.3	0
Salad dressing, blue cheese	1 tbsp	77	8	0.7	1.1	0
Salad dressing, caesar	1 tbsp	78	8.5	0.2	0.5	0
Salad dressing, coleslaw	1 tbsp	61	5.2	0.1	3.7	0
Salad dressing, french	1 tbsp	71	7	0.1	2.4	0
Salad dressing, honey dijon	1 tbsp	57.5	5	0.5	3	0.5
Salad dressing, italian	1 tbsp	43	4.2	0.1	1.5	0
Salad dressing, mayo-based	1 tbsp	57	4.9	0.1	3.5	0
Salad dressing, mayonnaise	1 tbsp	103	11.7	0	0	0
Salad dressing, peppercorn	1 tbsp	76	8.2	0.2	0.5	0
Salad dressing, ranch	1 tbsp	25	0	0	0	0
Salad dressing, russian	1 tbsp	76	7.8	0.2	1.6	0
Salad, chicken	6 oz.	420	33	45	11	1.5
Salad, egg	6 oz.	300	23	20	14	0.5
Salad, prima pasta	6 oz.	360	30	4.8	18	2.5
Salad, seafood w/ crab & shrimp	6 oz.	420	34	0	20	0
Salad, tuna	6 oz.	450	36	16	14	0
Salami, cooked, turkey	1 oz	37.7	2.3	0.7	0	0
Salami, dry, pork or beef	3 slices	104	8.1	6.3	1	0
Salami, italian pork	1 oz	119	10.4	6.1	0.3	0
Salsa, w/ oil	2 tbsp	40	3	0	8	0
Salsa, w/o oil	2 tbsp	15	0	0	3.5	0
Salt	1 tbsp	0	0	0	0	0
Sauce, alfredo	1/4 cup	120	11	15	3	2
Sauce, bbq	1 cup	188	4.5	4.5	32	3
Sauce, cheese	1 cup	479	36.3	25.1	13.3	0.2
Sauce, cranberry	1 cup	418	0.4	0.6	107.8	2.8
Sauce, hollandaise	1 cup	62	1.5	2.3	10.3	0.2
Sauce, honey mustard	1 tbsp	30	1	0	5	0
Sauce, marinara	1 cup	185	6	4.9	28.2	1
Sauce, salsa	1 cup	70	0.4	4	16.2	4.1
Sauce, soy	1 tbsp	10	0	0	0	0
Sauce, steak	1 tbsp	25	0	0	6	0
Sauce, teriyaki	1 tbsp	15	0	17	2	0
Sauce, tomato chili	1 cup	284	0.8	6.8	54	16.1
Sauce, worcestershire	1 cup	184	0	0	53.5	0
Sauerkraut	1/2 cup	25	0	1	5	4
Sausage, italian pork, raw	1 link	391	35.4	16.1	0.7	0
Sausage, pork	1 link	85	7.4	4.2	0	0
Sausage, smoked linked, pork	1 link	265	21.6	15.1	1.4	0
Sausage, turkey	1 link	0	0	0	0	0
Savory, ground	1 tsp	4	0.1	0.1	1	0.6
Scallops	1 scallop	26	0.2	5	0.7	0
Seaweed, dried	1 oz.	50	0	0	13	0
Sesame seeds, dried	1 tbsp	52	4.5	1.6	2.1	1.1
Shallots	1 tbsp, chopped	7	0	0.3	1.7	0
Shortening	1 tbsp	113	12.8	0	0	0
Shrimp, mixed species, raw	1 medium piece	6	0.1	1.2	0.1	0
Snacks, cheese puffs or twists	1 oz.	157	9.7	2.1	15.2	0.3

NUTRITIONAL INFORMATION

Nutrition values for fat, protein, carbohydrates, and fiber are listed in grams per serving.
Serving sizes and values are approximate.

FOOD ITEM	Serving Size	Cal.	Fat	Protein	Carbs	Fiber
S (cont.)						
Soda, club	12 fl oz.	0	0	0	0	0
Soda, cream	12 fl oz.	252	0	0	65.7	0
Soda, diet cola	12 fl oz.	0	0	0	0	0
Soda, ginger-ale	12 fl oz.	166	0	0	42.8	0
Soda, lemon-lime	12 fl oz.	196	0	0	51.1	0
Soda, regular, w/ caffeine	12 fl oz.	155	0	0.2	39.8	0
Soda, regular, w/o caffeine	12 fl oz.	207	0	0.2	52.9	0
Soda, root beer	12 fl oz.	202	0	0	52.3	0
Soda, tonic water	12 fl oz.	166	0	0	42.9	0
Soup, beef broth	1 cup	29	0	5.3	1.7	0
Soup, beef stroganoff	1 cup	235	11	12.2	21.6	1.4
Soup, beef vegetable	1 cup	82	1.9	2.9	13.1	0.5
Soup, chicken broth	1 cup	39	1.3	4.9	0.9	0
Soup, chicken noodle	1 cup	75	2.4	4	9.3	0.7
Soup, chicken vegetable	1 cup	75	2.8	3.6	8.5	1
Soup, chicken w/ dumplings	1 cup	96	5.5	5.6	6	0.5
Soup, clam chowder	1 cup	95	2.8	4.8	12.4	1.5
Soup, cream of chicken	1 cup	117	7.3	3.4	9.2	0.2
Soup, cream of mushroom	1 cup	129	8.9	2.3	9.3	0.5
Soup, cream of potato	1 cup	149	6.4	5.7	17	0.5
Soup, minestrone	1 cup	82	2.5	4.2	11.2	1
Soup, split-pea w/ham	1 cup	190	4.4	10.3	27.9	2.3
Soup, tomato	1 cup	161	6	6.1	22.3	2.7
Soup, vegetarian	1 cup	72	1.9	2.1	11.9	0.5
Sour cream	1 tbsp	26	2.5	0.4	0.5	0
Sour cream, fat free	1 tbsp	9	0	0.3	1.8	0
Sour cream, reduced fat	1 tbsp	22	1.7	0.8	0.8	0
Soy milk	1 cup	127	4.7	10.9	12	3.2
Soy protein isolate	1 oz	96	1	22.9	2.1	1.6
Soybeans, green, cooked	1 cup	254	11.5	22.2	19.8	7.6
Soybeans, nuts, roasted	1/4 cup	194	9.2	17	14	3.4
Soyburger	1 patty	125	4.1	12.5	9.3	3.2
Spaghetti, cooked	1 cup	197	0.9	6.6	39.6	2.4
Spaghetti, spinach, cooked	1 cup	182	0.8	6.4	36.6	2.4
Spaghetti, whole-wheat, cooked	1 cup	174	0.7	7.4	37.1	6.3
Spinach	1 cup	7	0.1	0.9	1.1	0.7
Squab, boneless, raw	1 squab	585	47.4	36.8	0	0
Squab, skinless, raw	1 squab	239	12.6	29.4	0	0
Squash, summer	1 cup, sliced	18	0.2	1.4	3.8	1.2
Squash, winter	1 cup, cubed	39	0.2	1.1	10	1.7
Squid, mixed species, raw	1 oz	26	0.4	4.4	0.9	0
Stock, beef	1 cup	31	0.2	4.7	2.9	0
Stock, chicken	1 cup	86	2.9	6	8.5	0
Stock, fish	1 cup	40	1.9	5.3	0	0
Strawberries	1 cup	49	0.5	1	11.7	3
Succotash	1 piece	0	0	0	0	0
Sugar, brown	1 tsp	12	0	0	3.1	0
Sugar, granulated	1 tsp	16	0	0	4.2	0
Sugar, maple	1 tsp	11	0	0	2.7	0
Sugar, powdered	1 tsp	10	0	0	2.5	0

NUTRITIONAL INFORMATION

Nutrition values for fat, protein, carbohydrates, and fiber are listed in grams per serving.
Serving sizes and values are approximate.

FOOD ITEM	Serving Size	Cal.	Fat	Protein	Carbs	Fiber
S (cont.)						
Sunflower seeds	1 tbsp	45	10	4	1.5	5
Sweet potato	1 cup, cubed	114,	0.1	2.1	26.8	4
Syrup, chocolate	1 tbsp	66.5	1.7	0.8	11.9	0.5
Syrup, dark corn	1 tbsp	57	0	0	15.5	0
Syrup, grenadine	1 tbsp	53	0	0	13.3	0
Syrup, light corn	1 tbsp	59	0	0	15.9	0
Syrup, maple	1 tbsp	52	0	0	13.4	0
Syrup, pancake	1 tbsp	47	0	0	12.3	0.1
T						
Taco shell, hard	1 shell	55	3	2	6	0
Tangerines	1 large	52	0.3	0.8	13.1	1.8
Tarragon, dried	1 tsp	2	0	0.1	0.3	0
Tea, instant	1 cup	2	0	0.1	0.4	0
Thyme	1 tsp	1	0	0	0.2	0.1
Thyme, dried	1 tsp	3	0.1	0.1	0.6	0.4
Tofu, firm	1/2 cup	183	11	19.9	5.4	2.9
Tofu, fried	1 piece	35	2.6	2.2	1.4	0.5
Tofu, soft	1/2 cup	75.5	4.6	8.1	2.2	0.2
Tomato juice, canned, with salt	6 fl oz	31	0.1	1.4	7.7	0.7
Tomato juice, canned, without salt	6 fl oz	30	0.1	1.2	7.8	0.7
Tomato paste, canned	1/2 cup	107	0.6	5.7	24.8	5.9
Tomato sauce, canned	1 cup	78	0.6	3.2	18.1	3.7
Tomatoes, canned, crushed	1 cup	82	0.7	4.2	18.6	4.8
Tomatoes, green	1 cup, chopped	41	0.4	2.2	9.2	2
Tomatoes, orange	1 cup, chopped	25	0.3	1.8	5	1.4
Tomatoes, red	1 cup, chopped	32	0.4	1.6	7.1	2.2
Tomatoes, sun-dried	1 cup, chopped	139	1.6	7.6	30.1	6.6
Toppings, butterscotch or caramel	2 tbsp	103	0	0.6	27	0.4
Toppings, marshmallow crème	2 tbsp	132	0.1	0.3	32.3	0
Toppings, nuts in syrup	2 tbsp	184	9	1.8	23.8	0.9
Toppings, pineapple	2 tbsp	106	0	0	27.9	0.2
Toppings, strawberry	2 tbsp	107	0	0.1	27.8	0.3
Tortilla chips, plain	1 oz.	142	7.4	1.9	17.8	1.8
Tortilla, corn	1 tortilla	45	0.5	2	9	3
Tortilla, flour	1 tortilla	160	3	18	28	3
Trail mix	1/4 cup	173.2	11	5	16.8	3
Turkey, deli sliced, white meat	1 oz.	30	1	5	0.5	0
Turkey, back, skinless, boneless, raw	1/2 back	180	5.3	31	0	0
Turkey, breast, boneless, raw	1/2 breast	541	11.5	102.9	0	0
Turkey, breast, skinless, boneless, raw	1/2 breast	433	2.5	95.9	0	0
Turkey, dark meat, boneless, raw	1/2 turkey	686	25.5	106.7	0	0
Turkey, dark meat, skinless, boneless, raw	1/2 turkey	532	12.8	98	0	0
Turkey, leg, boneless, raw	1 leg	412	12.5	70.3	0	0
Turkey, leg, skinless, boneless, raw	1 leg	355	7.8	67	0	0
Turkey, wing, boneless, raw	1 wing	204	9.9	26.7	0	0
Turkey, wing, skinless, boneless, raw	1 wing	95	1	20.2	0	0
Turkey, young hen, back, boneless, raw	1/2 back	650	47.5	52.2	0	0
Turkey, young hen, breast, boneless, raw	1/2 breast	1460	72.5	189	0	0
Turkey, young hen, dark meat, boneless, raw	1/2 turkey	1056	39.6	163	0	0

NUTRITIONAL INFORMATION

Nutrition values for fat, protein, carbohydrates, and fiber are listed in grams per serving. Serving sizes and values are approximate.

FOOD ITEM	Serving Size	Cal.	Fat	Protein	Carbs	Fiber
T (cont.)						
Turkey, young hen, leg, boneless, raw	1 leg	991	49.2	127.7	0	0
Turkey, young hen, wing, boneless, raw	1 wing	470	31.1	44.6	0	0
Turkey, young tom, back, boneless, raw	1/2 back	938	58.4	96.8	0	0
Turkey, young tom, breast, boneless, raw	1/2 breast	2701	113.4	392.9	0	0
Turkey, young tom, dark meat, boneless, raw	1/2 turkey	1884	63	307	0	0
Turkey, young tom, leg, boneless, raw	1 leg	1740	78.2	241.1	0	0
Turkey, young tom, wing, boneless, raw	1 wing	654	39	71.2	0	0
Turnip greens	1 cup, chopped	18	0.2	0.8	3.9	1.8
Turnips	1 cup, cubed	36	0.1	1.2	8.4	2.3
V						
Vanilla extract	1 tbsp	37	0	0	1.6	0
Veal, breast, raw	1 oz	59	4.2	5	0	0
Veal, cubed, raw	1 oz	31	0.7	5.7	0	0
Veal, ground, raw	1 oz	41	1.9	5.5	0	0
Veal, leg, raw	1 oz	33	0.9	5.9	0	0
Veal, loin, raw	1 oz	46	2.6	5.4	0	0
Veal, rib, raw	1 oz	46	2.6	5.3	0	0
Veal, shank, raw	1 oz	32	1	5.4	0	0
Veal, shoulder, arm, raw	1 oz	37	1.5	5.5	0	0
Veal, shoulder, blade, raw	1 oz	37	1.5	5.5	0	0
Veal, shoulder, whole, raw	1 oz	37	1.5	5.5	0	0
Veal, sirloin, raw	1 oz	43	2.2	5.4	0	0
Vegetable juice	8 fl oz.	50	0	2	12	2
Vinegar	1 tbsp	2	0	0	0.8	0
W						
Waffles, plain	1 waffle	218	10.6	5.9	24.7	0
Walnuts	1 oz. (14 halves)	185	18.5	4.3	3.9	1.9
Wasabi root	1 cup, sliced	142	0.8	6.2	30.6	10.1
Water chestnuts, chinese	1/2 cup, sliced	60	0.1	0.9	14.8	1.9
Watercress	1 cup, chopped	4	0	0.8	0.4	0.2
Watermelon	1 cup, diced	46	0.2	0.9	11.5	0.6
Wheat bran	1 cup	125	2.5	9	37.4	24.8
Wheat flour, whole grain	1 cup	407	2.2	16.4	87.1	14.6
Wheat germ	1 cup	414	11.2	26.6	59.6	15.2
Whipped cream	1 cup	154	13.3	1.9	7.5	0
Wine, cooking	1 tsp	2	0	0	0.3	0
Wine, red	3-1/2 oz. glass	74	0	0.2	1.8	0
Wine, rose	3-1/2 oz. glass	73	0	0.2	1.4	0
Wine, white	3-1/2 oz. glass	70	0	0.1	0.8	0
Yam	1 cup, cubed	177	0.3	2.3	41.8	6.1
Yeast, active, dry	1 tsp	12	0.2	1.5	1.5	0.8
Yogurt, fruit, low-fat	8 oz. container	118	0.3	5.5	23.8	0
Yogurt, fruit, whole milk	8 oz. container	250	6	9	38	0
Yogurt, plain, low-fat	8 oz. container	110	4	7.9	7	0
Yogurt, plain, whole milk	8 oz. container	138	7.4	12	10.6	0
Z						
Zucchini	1 medium	45	0	2	10	1